M000025175

Ultrasound Exam Review

SONOGRAPHER'S SELF-ASSESSMENT GUIDE

Second Edition

MARVEEN CRAIG, R.D.M.S.

with two contributors

J. B. Lippincott Company
Philadelphia

Acquisitions Editor: Andrew Allen
Sponsoring Editor: Maureen Mohan
Production Editor: Virginia Barishek
Interior Designer: Textbook Writers Associates
Cover Designer: Tom Jackson
Production: Textbook Writers Associates
Compositor: Circle Graphics
Prepress: Jay's Publishers Services, Inc.
Printer/Binder: R.R. Donnelley & Sons Company/Crawfordsville
Color Insert Printer: Walsworth Publishing

Second Edition

Copyright © 1994, by J. B. Lippincott Company.
Copyright © 1985, by J. B. Lippincott Company. All rights reserved. No part of this book
may be used or reproduced in any manner whatsoever without written permission except
for brief quotations embodied in critical articles and reviews. Printed in the United States of
America. For information write J. B. Lippincott Company, 227 East Washington Square,
Philadelphia, Pennsylvania 19106.

6 5 4 3 2 1

Library of Congress Cataloging-in-Publication Data

Craig, Marveen.
    Ultrasound exam review : sonographer's self-assessment guide / Marveen Craig ; with
two contributors. — [2nd ed.]
        p.   cm.
    Includes bibliographical references.
    ISBN 0-397-55021-9
    1. Diagnosis, Ultrasonic—Examinations, questions, etc.
    I. Title.
    [DNLM: 1. Ultrasonography—examination questions. WB 18 C886u 1994]
    RC78.7.U4C7 1994
    616.07′543′076—dc20
    DNLM/DLC
    for Library of Congress   93-41354
                                                                                CIP

Any procedure or practice described in this book should be applied by the health-care
practitioner under appropriate supervision in accordance with professional standards of
care used with regard to the unique circumstances that apply in each practice situation.
Care has been taken to confirm the accuracy of information presented and to describe
generally accepted practices. However, the authors, editors, and publisher cannot accept any
responsibility for errors or omissions or for any consequences from application of the
information in this book and make no warranty express or implied, with respect to the
contents of the book.

Every effort has been made to ensure drug selections and dosages are in accordance with
current recommendations and practice. Because of ongoing research, changes in
government regulations and the constant flow of information on drug therapy, reactions and
interactions, the reader is cautioned to check the package insert for each drug for
indications, dosages, warnings and precautions, particularly if the drug is new or
infrequently used.

"Let knowledge grow from more to more"
Tennyson

To my son,
Greg Lawrence,
who has brought his special blend
of artistry and perfectionism
to every one of my ultrasound endeavors
. . . thank you.

Consultants/Contributors

JOHN C. POPE, III, B.S., P.A.C., R.D.M.S., R.D.C.S.

Affiliate Clinical Instructor
Physicians Assistant Department
Medical College of Georgia
Director, Echocardiography Laboratory
Cardiovascular Associates of Augusta
Augusta, Georgia

DENISE LEVY, R.T., R.D.M.S., R.V.T.

Consultant (formerly Supervisor)
Vascular Center
Good Samaritan Hospital
San Jose, California

Preface

In the field of diagnostic ultrasonography, the past eight years have seen continuation of the trend toward rapidly changing and expanding technology and its demand for an accompanying body of knowledge. To meet our obligations, the second edition of *Ultrasound Exam Review* has been completely rewritten and a vascular section has been added. There are over 100 more questions, and both instructors and students of diagnostic medical sonography programs were solicited to provide information for the "Cases and Questions" sections. Many more ultrasound images appear, and are included in every chapter, and, for the first time, color images are presented. Finally, we have placed more emphasis on deductive reasoning. This approach to revision is in keeping with our original goal: to provide a concise yet current review of the fundamentals of diagnostic medical sonography.

The initiation and publication of this project owes a great deal to the tenacity of my editor, Andrew Allen, who helped and encouraged me at many stages of the process.

Our new edition is enhanced by the contributions of John Charles Pope and Denise Moulton Levy, who patiently consulted with and educated me and skillfully executed the echocardiographic and vascular sections.

From its inception to its completion, the project could not have taken place without the supportive and loving environment provided by my husband, Walter, and the encouragement and understanding of my family and friends.

All that remains is to thank you, the readers, for enthusiastically supporting the first edition of *Ultrasound Exam Review*. With the new edition we hope to once again meet our goal of providing student and registry-bound sonographers with an up-to-date, convenient, self-assessment resource.

Marveen Craig, R.D.M.S.

Acknowledgments

It is a pleasure to acknowledge the contributions of many new colleagues—the instructors and students of several leading diagnostic medical sonography programs. They accepted my challenge to take part in shaping a self-assessment book designed for their own use, and in the process, added immeasurably not only to this edition but to my hopes for the future of sonography.

I wish to thank them collectively, as well as crediting them individually within the text, for the cases and questions they so graciously provided.

Community College of Allegheny
Diagnostic Medical Sonography Program
Monroeville, Pennsylvania
Program Director: Lynn Gigandet, R.D.M.S., Ms.Ed.
Students: Anita Bowser, Lisa Elbert, Bonnie Kazior, and Susan Ley

Johns Hopkins Hospital
Diagnostic Medical Sonography Program
Baltimore, Maryland
Program Coordinator: Jan Bloomer, R.T., R.D.M.S.
Instructors: Steven Herman, B.S., R.D.M.S. and Patricia Lucas
Students: Noelle Blair, Pat Colombo, Joanne Cramer, Yvonne Hoeflich, Linda Lang, Jay Milio, James Pennington, Patricia Revaj, Lance Silwick, Gale White, and Nancy Wityk

Ochsner Medical Foundation
Diagnostic Medical Sonography Program
New Orleans, Louisiana
Program Director: Benita D. Barthel, R.T.R., R.D.M.S.
Students: Dixie Alexander, Alicia Fernandez, Michelle Guillory, and Jeanie Marchese

Orange Coast College
Diagnostic Medical Sonography Program
Costa Mesa, California
Program Director: Joan M. Clasby, R.T., R.D.M.S.
Students: Laura Arteaga, Jo Addington, Stacey Beck, Michelle Bolitho, Jennifer Cooper-Wilson, Linda Foreman, Gail Gould, Janie Hay, Laura Hodge, Mark Houck, Carmen Hunn, Sheila Lind, Carrie Lundy, Ed Marsh, Laura McNaughton, Cheryl Powell, Lynda Ranson, Carrie Robbins, Kathy Shupe, Amy Stillman, Angela Tyvog, and Marsha Wolfson

Palm Beach Community College
Diagnostic Medical Sonography Program
Palm Beach Gardens, Florida
Program Director: Sandra M. Karol, M.A., R.D.M.S., R.T.
Students: Linda Novick, R.T. and Richard Lane

Rhode Island School of Diagnostic Medical Sonography
Rhode Island Hospital
Providence, Rhode Island
Program Director: Jack P. Grusmark, R.D.M.S.
Students: Kris Kuros, Kristine Mooney, Janice St. Jean, and Kathy Toledo

St. Francis Hospital
School of Diagnostic Medical Sonography
Milwaukee, Wisconsin
Program Director: Stephanie Maass, R.T., R.D.M.S.
Students: Dayna Landru and Tracy Pfizenmaier

State University of New York (SUNY)
Diagnostic Medical Imaging Program
College of Health Related Professions
Brooklyn, New York
Program Director: Mimi C. Berman, Ph.D., R.D.M.S.
Instructor: Joyce Miller, R.T., R.D.M.S.
Students: Yansheng Wei and Judy Schwartz

University of Iowa Hospitals and Clinics
Diagnostic Medical Sonography Program
Iowa City, Iowa
Program Director: Marilyn Holland, R.D.M.S.
Instructor: Stephanie Ellingson, R.T.R., R.D.M.S.

I also wish to acknowledge two members of the West Virginia Diagnostic Ultrasound Society, Kathy Dopson, R.D.M.S. and Adele Hoffman, R.D.M.S., for graciously providing images from their study of an ovarian ectopic pregnancy.

Special thanks is owed to William G. Hayden, M.D., Redwood City, California, Drs. David E. Smith and Richard W. Starett of San Jose, California, Advanced Technology Laboratories, Bothell, Washington, and Quantum Medical Systems, Inc., Division of Siemens, Issaquah, Washington, for providing case studies to the vascular section.

Contents

Contents

Marveen Craig: *Ultrasound Exam Review*, © 1994 J. B. Lippincott Co.

1

Physics

OBJECTIVES

Diagnostic ultrasonography, unlike many forms of imaging, requires constant use of the applied physical principles of sound in the creation and interpretation of ultrasound images. Therefore, sonographers must possess a fundamental knowledge of the physical principles of sound, a detailed understanding of current ultrasonic instruments, and an appreciation of the complex interactions of ultrasound in a variety of biologic tissues. This chapter attempts to integrate those essentials and present them in a way that will stimulate registry-bound sonographers, as well as educational specialists, in search of additional teaching aids.

QUESTIONS

Directions

Each of the questions or incomplete statements is followed by several answers or completions. Select the best answer(s) in each case. In the matching sections, answers should be used only once, unless otherwise stated.

1. The transmission of ultrasound is highly dependent on a medium's _____ and _____.
   A. density; compressibility
   B. compressibility; acoustic impedance
   C. specular quality; weight
   D. size; shape

2. Soft-tissue echoes must be amplified before they can be displayed. This action is accomplished by the:
   A. receiver.
   B. frequency analyzer.
   C. RF amplifier.
   D. initial gain.

3. In order to produce a single frame, or picture, on the average television monitor, the electron beam sweeps across the screen from right to left. It requires _____ of these sweeps (lines) to produce a single frame.
   A. 225
   B. 250
   C. 525
   D. 552

4. The thickness in tissue (in cm) required to reduce the intensity of the sound beam by half is called the:
   A. half power level.
   B. half value layer.
   C. subtraction layer.
   D. half tone layer.

5. Which of the following are characteristics of sound?
   A. Waves of frequency between 20 Hz and 20 kHz
   B. A mechanical disturbance that travels through a medium at constant speed
   C. Electromagnetic energy
   D. A and B

6. Most diagnostic ultrasound transducers are focused by:
   A. spherical elements or lenses.
   B. convex elements.
   C. modulators.
   D. A and B

7. Wave fronts advance at a fixed velocity determined by:
   A. frequency.
   B. the heat generated.
   C. the material and medium.
   D. duration.

8. Which of the following statements about axial resolution is (are) correct?
   A. Proportional to pulse duration
   B. Increases with higher frequency
   C. If frequency increases, wavelength decreases
   D. All of the above

9. Identify the types of signal processing presented in Figure 1-1.

   1. ____   A. RF

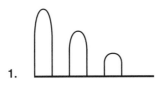

1.

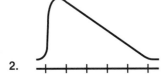

2.

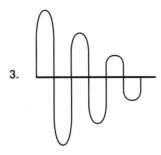

3.

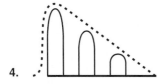

4.

Figure 1-1. Examples of signal processing.

2. ____   B. Demodulated
3. ____   C. Enveloped
4. ____   D. Video form

10. The amplitude range of echoes in a typical ultrasound examination is approximately _____ decibels (dB).
    A. 25
    B. 40
    C. 60
    D. 75

11. Which of the following state-

ments are *not* characteristic of Doppler ultrasound?
    A. Records frequency shift and may produce audible signals
    B. Produces aliasing at the Nyberg frequency
    C. May utilize dual transducers
    D. Employs pulsed wave techniques

12. Electronically varying the amplification of sound as the beam travels deeper into the body describes:
    A. attenuation.
    B. receiver gain.
    C. TGC.
    D. demodulation.

Match the following to numbers 13–20.

    A. Pulsed average
    B. Temporal average
    C. Intensity
    D. Radiation force
    E. W/cm^2
    F. Temporal peak
    G. Temporal intensity
    H. I

13. ____ The concentration of power within a sound beam
14. ____ The maximum intensity of a sound beam that occurs in space and time
15. ____ The average throughout the entire duration of a pulse
16. ____ The maximum intensity of an ultrasound beam at any point in time

17. ___ The unit used to measure power (intensity)

18. ___ A small steady force produced when sound beams strike reflecting or absorbing interfaces

19. ___ Intensity averaged over the entire pulse repetition period

20. ___ The average throughout both transmitting and receiving activities

21. Identify the parts of the ultrasound beam represented in Figure 1-2.

   1. ___   A. Focal point
   2. ___   B. Beam divergence
   3. ___   C. Focal length
   4. ___   D. Crystal
   5. ___   E. Focal zone

Match the correct terms and definitions for numbers 22–25.

   A. Absorption
   B. Specular reflector
   C. Refraction
   D. Impedance
   E. Reflection
   F. Resolution
   G. Scattering
   H. Compression

22. ___ Greatest source of attenuation in tissues

23. ___ Result of surface irregularities of 1 wavelength or less

24. ___ Plane boundary perpendicular to sound propagation

25. ___ Change in the direction of an incident beam

26. The use of higher frequencies results in ___ resolution and ___ attenuation.
   A. increased; decreased
   B. increased; increased
   C. decreased; increased
   D. decreased; decreased

27. In a diagnostic ultrasound setting, the total pulse duration is ___ the period of pulse repetition frequency.
   A. equal to
   B. greater than
   C. less than
   D. none of the above

28. Ultrasound attenuates an average of ___ dB/cm of travel for each megahertz of frequency.
   A. 1
   B. 0.75
   C. 1/2
   D. 0.25

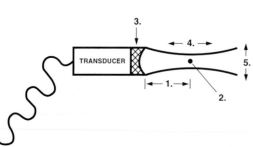

Figure 1-2. Components of an ultrasound beam.

29. Spherical sound waves are emitted from small elements of the transducer area in 1-wavelength increments that reinforce and develop into a plane wave front. This phenomenon is known as:
    A. Ohm's law.
    B. Young's modulus.
    C. Huygen's principle.
    D. Hurler's law.

30. Phased-array transducers can be identified by their:
    A. scan line of 1 line/mm.
    B. sector shape.
    C. scan line of 1 line/degree.
    D. B and C

31. Immediately adjacent to the face of a transducer the ultrasound wave front is collimated and well defined. This area is known as the:
    A. Fresnel zone or near field.
    B. Fraunhofer zone or far field.
    C. focal zone.
    D. A and B

32. The distortion of crystal shape by an electrical stimulus and the generation of an electrical signal by mechanical distortion of the crystal describes the:
    A. dead zone of the transducer.
    B. piezoelectric (pressure-electric) effect.
    C. transducer's Q factor.
    D. all of the above

33. Particle movement along the direction of energy flow is referred to as a:
    A. reflection.
    B. longitudinal wave.
    C. convex wave.
    D. transverse wave.

34. The intensity of sound is greatest in:
    A. the Fresnel zone.
    B. the Fraunhoffer zone.
    C. the amplifier.
    D. the focal zone.

35. The term _____ describes the fact that structures lying behind weakly reflecting interfaces will appear more prominent than they really are.
    A. shadowing
    B. enhancement
    C. reverberation
    D. registration

36. A transducer that contains damping material with an acoustic impedance very similar to that of the crystal element will produce:
    A. considerable ringing.
    B. a highly damped waveform.
    C. increased oscillations.
    D. expanded envelopes of ultrasonic vibration.

37. The angle of refraction depends on the _____ of ultrasound in each medium.
    A. frequency
    B. velocity
    C. intensity
    D. duration

38. When the molecules of a medium are agitated vigorously, the ultrasound intensity will:
    A. increase.
    B. decrease.

C. be neutralized.
D. B and C

39. The degree of divergency of the far field is determined by _____ and _____.
A. diameter; wave front
B. transducer size; frequency
C. the near field; the far field
D. crystal thickness; frequency

Match the following list to numbers 40–50.

A. Acoustic speckle
B. Slice or section thickness
C. Refraction
D. Reverberation
E. Comet tail
F. Mirror image
G. Multipath
H. Side lobes
 I. Grating lobes
J. Propagation speed errors
K. Acoustic shadow

40. ____ Reflectors can be placed in improper positions on an image if sound travels at a speed other than 1540 m/s
41. ____ Waves changing direction when traveling from one medium to another can cause image placement on the screen in improper locations
42. ____ When the paths that the pulse travels to and from a reflector are of different lengths, the pulse may glance off a second structure on the way to or from the primary reflector
43. ____ An artifact produced by the interference of ultrasound wavelets

44. ____ A type of reverberation echo characterized by a linear series of bands (or a thin line of echoes) trailing off within an essentially echo-free area
45. ____ The appearance of reflections produced by structures above or below a beam's main axis
46. ____ A sound "bounce" off a strong reflector in its path that creates an incorrectly spaced, spurious second image
47. ____ Linear-array transducer production of off-axis acoustic waves as a result of the regular spacing of the active elements
48. ____ Divergence of some of the power in the main beam to produce "pockets" adjacent to the main beam
49. ____ Regularly repeated, parallel echoes produced by reflections from a strong reflector, usually close to the skin surface
50. ____ Absence of sound distal to a strong reflector

51. Which of the following parameters is (are) not considered part of a beam profile?
A. Intensity
B. Diameter
C. Housing
D. Focusing

52. Label Figure 1-3 using the following terms.

1. ____   A. Near gain
2. ____   B. Far gain

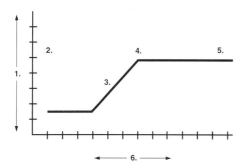

Figure 1-3. Time gain compensation curve.

3. ___   C. Slope
4. ___   D. Depth/time
5. ___   E. Amplitude
6. ___   F. Knee

53. The velocity of sound in the soft tissues of the body:
    A. is 1540 m/cm.
    B. ranges from 1480 to 1640 m/s.
    C. averages 1540 m/s.
    D. B and C

54. Distance can be computed by multiplying:
    A. time × intensity.
    B. velocity × intensity.
    C. time × velocity.
    D. round trip time/2 × 1450 m/s.

55. The percentage of reflected energy produced when a longitudinal ultrasound wave reaches a second material with different acoustic properties depends on:
    A. the acoustic mismatch.
    B. the density of one material.
    C. the amount of sound continuing on.
    D. all of the above

56. Axial resolution is equal to _____ of the spatial pulse length (SPL).
    A. $1/8$
    B. $1/4$
    C. $1/3$
    D. $1/2$

57. When scanning patients with excessive subcutaneous fat, the sonographer should _____ the start of the TGC curve.
    A. increase
    B. delay
    C. select a point approximately $1/2$ the patient's body thickness for
    D. select a point approximately $1/4$ the patient's body thickness for

58. Ultrasound waves moving through human tissue create alternating areas of increased and decreased pressure, which cause the formation of gas bubbles subject to cavitation. As the bubbles grow, they resonate and may produce:
    A. microstreaming.
    B. shock waves.
    C. molecular and cellular damage.
    D. all of the above

59. Color-flow imaging provides forward or reverse flow and intensity information in color while simultaneously providing two-dimensional images of structures adjacent to the vessels. A(n) _____ appears as a color that is different from those which correctly represent normal forward and reverse flow.

A. aliasing artifact
B. autocoloration artifact
C. autocorrelation artifact
D. fourier artifact

60. Compressed molecules within a medium will eventually return to a relaxed state. This process is called:
    A. reflection.
    B. attenuation.
    C. rarefaction.
    D. realignment.

61. To remove all air from between the face of the transducer and the patient's skin requires the use of various coupling media. Such media must be comparable to the acoustic impedance of soft tissue, which is approximately _____.
    A. 1.48
    B. 1.63
    C. 1.43
    D. 1.1540

62. How is the Q or quality factor of a transducer determined?
    A. The frequency is divided by the beamwidth
    B. The frequency is divided by the bandwidth
    C. The frequency is multiplied by the beamwidth
    D. The frequency is multiplied by the bandwidth

63. Which of the following statements about the decibel scale is (are) true?
    A. It can be used to compare intensities, and it is additive and subtractive.
    B. It is a logarithmic scale which provides a convenient way of compressing a wide range of intensities.
    C. It permits the use of negative decibel values to represent attenuation.
    D. all of the above

64. In comparing transducer bandwidth, it is important to note that a narrow-bandwidth crystal will vibrate for a(n) _____ period of time, whereas a wide-bandwidth crystal tends to ring for a(n) _____ period.
    A. long; shorter
    B. short; longer
    C. finite; infinite
    D. intermittently; continuously

65. Interfaces that are _____ with respect to the wavelength of the sound beam are called *specular reflectors*.
    A. large and smooth
    B. small and rough
    C. slightly irregular
    D. greatly irregular

66. The percentage or fraction of time that an ultrasound system is producing a pulse or is transmitting sound is called the *duty factor* or *duty cycle*. The duty factor is equal to the _____ divided by the _____.
    A. pulse length; temporal average
    B. maximum value; minimum value
    C. pulse duration; pulse repetition period
    D. voltage; period

67. A/an _____ transducer consists of a series of concentric rings fired in rapid sequence.
    A. annular
    B. wobbler
    C. steered
    D. cylindrical

68. The mechanical energy extracted from a wave by absorption is converted into _____ within the medium.
    A. liquid
    B. viscosities
    C. heat
    D. null sound

69. Sound traveling 1540 m/s, emitted by a 3.5 MHz transducer, will have a wavelength of:
    A. 0.86 mm.
    B. 0.62 mm.
    C. 0.44 mm.
    D. 0.24 mm.

Match the following list to numbers 70–74.

    A. Hertz
    B. Property of reflection
    C. Piezoelectric
    D. Active element
    E. dB/cm/unit of fx

70. ____ Attenuation
71. ____ Cycles per second
72. ____ Acoustic impedance
73. ____ Transducer
74. ____ Quartz

75. Acoustic impedance is equal to:
    A. $Z = p/c$.
    B. $Z = pc$.

C. $Z = c/p$.
D. none of the above

76. Refraction of the ultrasound beam by the rectus muscles contributes to the production of a common artifact, the:
    A. reduction artifact.
    B. doubling artifact.
    C. ghost artifact.
    D. split artifact.

77. Choose the answers that correctly match the appropriate units and factors.

	λ	Hz	Speed	Intensity	Attenuation
A.	m/s	m/s²	Hz	J/cm²	MHz
B.	M	MHz	Hz/s	A/m²	W/s
C.	mm	MHz	m/s	W/cm²	dB
D.	m	MHz	m/s	dB	W

Match the appropriate formula to numbers 78–82.

    A. Number of cycles/pulse multiplied by the period
    B. Power at center of field/area at center of field
    C. Total power/total area
    D. Pulse duration/PRP
    E. Number of cycles × wavelength

78. ____ Duty factor
79. ____ Spatial pulse length
80. ____ Peak intensity
81. ____ Pulse duration
82. ____ Spatial average intensity

83. Which of the following is the transducer of choice for scanning a 1-mm lesion in the thyroid?
    A. 1–2.25 MHz
    B. 3.5 MHz

C. 5 MHz

D. 7.5–10 MHz

84. Pulse echo systems operate in the receive mode approximately _____% of each cycle.
   A. 9
   B. 9.9
   C. 99
   D. 100

85. With respect to artifacts, sonographers should:
   A. recognize and eliminate their presence.
   B. rotate the transducer 90 degrees and rescan.
   C. use the artifact as diagnostic information, if possible.
   D. all of the above

86. Ultrasound phantoms (such as the one presented in Fig. 1-4) are available to help sonographers measure such parameters as:
   A. transducer focus.
   B. tissue penetration.
   C. distance measurement accuracy.
   D. all of the above

87. Why are side lobe artifacts troublesome to sonographers?
   A. They falsely duplicate structures
   B. They prevent accurate measurements
   C. They simulate layered particulate material within cysts
   D. They create acoustic shadows

88. Which of the following is (are) not characteristics of annular phased array transducers?
   A. Provide selective transmit focus
   B. Receive-focus dependent on transmit focus
   C. Focus the beam in all planes
   D. Provide good images in obese patients

Match the following terms to numbers 89–93.
   A. apodization
   B. diameter
   C. focal length
   D. focus
   E. focal zone

89. The _____ is the distance from the transducer face to the narrowest portion of the beam pattern.

90. The _____ is the range of axial distances over which the beam pattern is sufficiently narrow to produce good image spatial resolution.

91. The transducer _____ gets stronger as aperture increases.

92. Increasing the transducer _____ reduces the extent of the focal zone.

93. _____ results in the reduction of beam pattern side lobe amplitude.

94. The AIUM standard 100-mm test object (see Fig. 1-4) is usually filled with medium that simulates 1540 m/s sound velocity. Match the type of test related to the internal targets.
   A. Beamwidth calibration
   B. Axial resolution

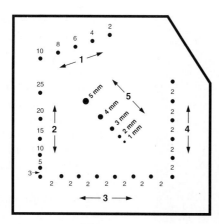

TEST OBJECT

Figure 1-4. AIUM standard 100-mm test object.

C. Vertical calibration
D. Dead zone measurement
E. Lateral resolution
1. ___ Group 1
2. ___ Column 2
3. ___ Row 3
4. ___ Column 4
5. ___ Group 5

95. Which of the following controls *does not* affect the amplification of echoes?
A. Slope rate
B. Attenuator
C. Energy output
D. Overall gain

Match the symbols to the prefixes in numbers 96–100.

96. ___ micro   A. k
97. ___ milli   B. M
98. ___ centi   C. μ
99. ___ kilo   D. m
100. ___ mega   E. c

101. Scan converters were adopted for use in sonography because of their ability to:
A. assign a shade of gray to each returning echo according to its decibel strength.
B. permit image manipulation, alteration, storage, or display.
C. permit the use of a television monitor for display.
D. all of the above

102. Increasing the transducer output decreases the resolution because:
A. it encourages artifacts.
B. higher intensity produces longer pulse lengths.
C. it alters beamwidth.
D. it upsets the TGC curve.

103. Which of the following statements regarding signal processing is *untrue*?
A. Preprocessing is done before storage in the scan converter
B. Preprocessing occurs before the information is digitized
C. Postprocessing occurs after data have been stored but prior to display
D. Requires signal compression

104. Spectral broadening is seen:
A. as a normal-appearing waveform.
B. if Doppler gain settings are too high.
C. when flow is turbulent.
D. A and B

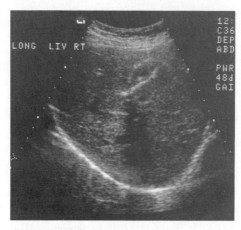

A

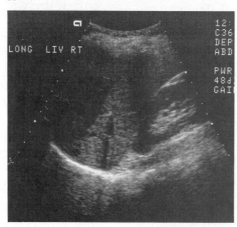

B

Figure 1-5. (*A*,*B*) Longitudinal scans of the right upper quadrant. (Courtesy of Steven Herman, BS, RDMS and James Pennington, Johns Hopkins Hospital, Baltimore, Maryland.)

105. The critical factor in determining frame rate, line density, and imaging depth is the:
    A. frequency.
    B. time.
    C. wavelength.
    D. CRT.

Numbers 106–108 refer to Figure 1-5*A*,*B*.

106. In these images, the "shadow" artifact is most likely the result of:
    A. refraction.
    B. range ambiguity.
    C. attenuation.
    D. section thickness.

107. If a sound propagation path to a reflector must partially pass through a structure whose speed of sound differs from 1540 m/s, the returning echoes are most likely to produce:
    A. focal banding.
    B. echo "position registration" artifact.
    C. slice thickness artifacts.
    D. distal "echo enlargement."

108. If the ultrasound intensity is sufficiently high and the molecular structure of the target tissue sufficiently loose, the violent molecular agitations can result in:
    A. ionization.
    B. thermal convection.
    C. cavitation.
    D. excitation.

Numbers 109–111 refer to Figure 1-6*A*,*B*.

109. In the images presented, the type of artifact seen near the diaphragm is most likely a _____ artifact.
    A. multipath
    B. refraction

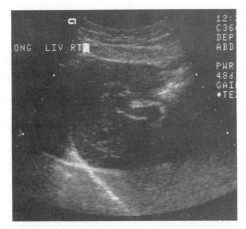

A

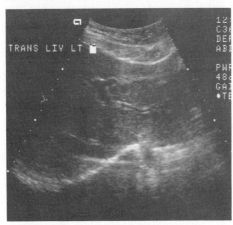

B

Figure 1-6. (*A*) Longitudinal scan of the right lobe of the liver. (*B*) Transverse scan of the left lobe of the liver. (Courtesy of Steven Herman, BS, RDMS and James Pennington, Johns Hopkins Hospital, Baltimore, Maryland.)

    C. mirror image
    D. reverberation

110. Which of the artifacts listed below is unrelated to the size, shape, or geometry of the ultrasound pulse?

    A. Lateral resolution
    B. Slice thickness
    C. Longitudinal resolution
    D. Mirror image

111. The anatomic structure associated with a mirror image artifact is:
    A. sometimes shallower on the image than in the body.
    B. always deeper on the image than in the body.
    C. sometimes the same depth on the image as in the body.
    D. never deeper on the image than in the body.

112. Which of the statements below is (are) *incorrect* regarding A-mode displays?
    A. Echo height proportional to strength
    B. Registers the distance of reflectors from the transducer
    C. Can demonstrate the difference between cysts and solid
    D. All of the above

113. B-mode, or brightness modulation, differs from the A-mode in that echo information is applied to the _____ of the oscilloscope.
    A. *X* axis
    B. *Y* axis
    C. *Z* axis
    D. *C* axis

114. Which of the following statements best defines the term *acoustic window*?
    A. An air-free surface

B. A homogeneous structure
C. An area through which sound passes unimpeded
D. An area consisting of only specular reflectors

Match the following terms to numbers 115–120.

A. Convex-curved arrays
B. Phased arrays
C. Linear-switched arrays
D. Annular-phased arrays
E. Compound-contact scanners
F. Water-path scanners

115. ___ An acoustic standoff or water path placed between the sweeping or steering mechanism and the patient

116. ___ Requires no beam steering because its design creates a sector image

117. ___ Elements fired in sequence to provide a two-dimensional image

118. ___ Incorporates a three-jointed arm for plotting position

119. ___ Provides identical dynamic extended focus in both vertical and horizontal planes

120. ___ Utilizes time delays in pulsing and receiving in order to focus and steer the beam

121. Piezoelectric materials exist in both natural and man-made states. The most common natural crystal is quartz; the most commonly used man-made crystal is:
A. PTP.
B. PZT.
C. BTP.
D. BZT.

ANSWERS

1. A. Medical diagnostic ultrasound must pass through a tissue medium. The transmission of sound depends on the medium's density and compressibility. Compressibility is a hard-to-measure property of matter: It is the ease with which matter can be deformed by an external force. The range of compressibility of matter is much greater than the range of density; therefore, compressibility is the principal determinant of ultrasound velocity.[2]

2. C. Most soft-tissue interfaces produce echoes that generate from 1 to 100 mv. These must be amplified before they can be displayed. This job is performed by the radio frequency (RF) amplifier, which multiplies the strength of the electric signal in a linear fashion; that is, every echo is amplified by the same amount.[1]

3. C. The electron beam is steered through a raster pattern, consisting of 525 horizontal lines, which sweeps horizontally across the screen, moves down one line, and sweeps again.[5]

4. B. When ultrasound is transmitted through tissue, it is reduced in intensity by energy absorption and dispersion. Together, these processes exponentially attenuate the beam. One consequence of this relationship is the analogous expression of half value layer. It can be shown that a 3-dB reduction in intensity is equivalent to a 50% reduction. Therefore, the thickness of tissue necessary to reduce beam intensity by 3 dB is the half value layer.[2,4]

5. D. Sound is a mechanical form of energy, which in contrast to electromagnetic energy requires a medium for propagation. By convention, sound consists of frequencies between 20 Hz and 20 kHz. Sound travels through a medium at a constant speed, and its velocity is measured in meters per second (m/s).[1,2,5,10,15]

6. D. Transducers are focused by either internal or external acoustic lenses or by shaping the crystal with a concave face, which causes the walls of the beam to converge.[16]

7. C. Sound advances at a constant speed through a medium. For practical considerations, the velocity (or speed) of ultrasound in biologic tissues is dependent on the physical properties of the tissue (material and medium) and is independent of the frequency.[10,15]

8. D. Axial resolution is the ability to resolve closely spaced interfaces lying along the path, or axis, of the sound beam. It is affected by

pulse length and influenced by frequency, since axial resolution can be no better than one wavelength. As frequency increases, wavelength decreases, and therefore, resolution increases. Azimuthal resolution refers to lateral, not axial, resolution.[1, 4, 16]

9. 1. B, 2. D, 3. A, 4. C

Once an ultrasound signal is received, it must be processed and converted into a form that can be displayed. The amplified RF waveform (A) of the electric signal produced by the returning echo is a sine wave. The negative portion of the wave cannot be used by the display system and is eliminated by the process of demodulation (B). The three peaks of the signal are converted to one peak (C), which converts the RF waveform into a video signal in the process known as *enveloping*. The video form signal (D) is then electronically manipulated in one or more ways to improve the appearance of the displayed image.[1, 10]

10. C. Although transmitters and receivers are able to handle a wide range of echo strengths, display systems are much more limited. The amplitude range of echoes in a typical ultrasound examination is about 60 dB; however, the best display systems can accept only up to a 25-dB range. Consequently, the video amplifier is used to compress the 60-dB range of incoming signals to a 25-dB range.[1]

11. B. The Doppler effect, or Doppler shift, is a change in the frequency of sound as a result of motion between the sound source and the receiver. Doppler shifts, which can be made audible, result from sound bouncing off of red blood cells. There are two major forms of Doppler currently used in medical diagnosis: continuous- and pulsed-wave techniques. Continuous-wave Doppler employs two crystals in the transducer (one receiver and one transmitter); pulsed-wave Doppler uses only one crystal but alternates between sending and receiving. Pulsed-wave Doppler is unable to measure high velocities correctly; instead, high velocities appear as a negative. This is called *aliasing*. The Nyquist frequency (or limit at which aliasing occurs) is equal to one-half the pulse-repetition frequency (PRF).[4–6]

12. C. The deeper an echoing structure is from the transducer, the more attenuation an echo reflecting from that structure will experience before being received back at the probe. The method of correcting for the attenuation of sound in tissues is called *time gain compensation (TGC)*, or swept gain.[4, 10, 16]

13. C   17. E

14. H   18. D

15. A   19. G

16. F   20. B[1, 4, 6, 10, 15]

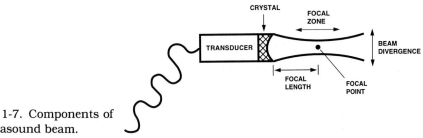

Figure 1-7. Components of
an ultrasound beam.

21. 1. C, 2. A, 3. D, 4. E, 5. B (See Fig. 1-7.)[1, 2, 6, 15]

22. A

23. G

24. B

25. C[1, 15]

26. B. Many factors influence resolution: focusing, frequency, pulse
    length, transducer geometry, etc. However, it should be noted that
    as frequency increases, tissue attenuation increases, and the pene-
    tration of the beam into the body decreases.[16]

27. C. The crystal of a transducer must act as both a transmitter and
    a receiver of sound. Therefore, the optimal situation occurs when a
    very short pulse of sound is emitted from the crystal, and the crys-
    tal spends a long time in waiting for returning echoes.[4, 16]

28. A. On average, an ultrasound beam traveling through human soft
    tissue will be attenuated 1 decibel (dB) per centimeter per mega-
    hertz (1 dB/cm/MHz).[1]

29. C. Simply stated, Huygen's principle means that a sound source
    that is very large compared with the wavelength can be thought of

as the sum of many point sources of sound that compose the single large source. Each point will emit waves in concentric rings. The farther the rings travel from the transducer, the more parallel they become, resulting in a more uniform beam.[2, 4, 16]

30. D. Phased-array scanning can usually be identified by the sector-shaped view it generates compared with the rectangular field of view generated by most linear-array transducer assemblies. Sonographers can often select the scan line, image frame rates, and the depth of scan with both types of transducers, since they are interdependent. A minimum acceptable scan line rate is 1 line/mm for linear arrays and 1 line/degree for phased arrays.[2]

31. D. When a circular crystal transducer emits a sound beam, the beam initially remains cylindrical along the direction of the beam axis. After traveling some distance, however, the beam begins to diverge. The area before the point of divergence is described as the *near field* or *Fresnel zone*, and the area comprising the diverging portion of the beam is the *far field* or *Fraunhofer zone*.[10]

32. B. Transducer operation is based on the piezoelectric (pressure-electric) effect. This effect occurs when certain materials (piezoelectric crystals) distort when an electrical signal is impressed across their short axis. By very rapidly reversing the polarity of this electrical signal, say with megahertz frequency, the piezoelectric crystal will respond accordingly, emitting sound at the megahertz level.[1, 2, 4, 16]

33. B. When a sound beam is applied to a medium, it causes the particles of the medium to vibrate, transmitting vibrations from particle to particle via their elastic connections. The most important vibration is the back-and-forth motion along the longitudinal axis of the beam, which creates longitudinal waves.[9, 10, 16]

34. D. The intensity of sound within a particular portion of the beam varies. The focal zone of the beam contains the most concentrated area of sound intensity.[16]

35. B. Image enhancement occurs when some of the superficial tissues have very low attenuation and the echo signals from some of the deeper tissues are overcompensated by the TGC system.[10] Structures that allow the sound to pass unimpeded give the appearance of enhanced transmission behind the mass. This quality is characteristic of fluid-filled or cystic structures. To accurately characterize the structures' internal nature, it is important to assess what hap-

pens to the sound as it passes through the structure under investigation.[16]

36. B. Damping materials are employed to limit the ringing of the pulse.[4,6]

37. B. The angle of refraction depends on the velocity of ultrasound in each medium. When an ultrasonic beam interacts at an interface between two tissues, some of the ultrasound will be transmitted across the interface and some will be reflected. If the acoustic impedances of the two tissues differ greatly, most of the ultrasound will be reflected and very little will be transmitted. If the tissues are very similar and have nearly equal acoustic impedances, more of the ultrasound will be transmitted.[2,10]

38. A. Ultrasound intensity increases when the molecules of the medium are agitated more vigorously. The energy imparted to these tissues is the intensity of the ultrasound and is expressed as energy per unit area (milliwatts per square centimeter, or mW/cm^2).[2,9,14]

39. B. The degree of divergency in the far field is determined by transducer size and operating frequency according to the following forumla:

$$\sin 0 - \frac{1.22}{D}$$

where 0 is the angle of divergence.[2]

40. J

41. C

42. G

43. A

44. E

45. B

46. F

47. I

48. H

49. D

50. K[4-9]

51. C. Manufacturers provide a printout of the beam profiles of each transducer. This is a plot of the intensity of sound at various distances from the transducer face. It displays not only sound intensity but also the width of the beam at specific distances from the transducer.[6, 16]

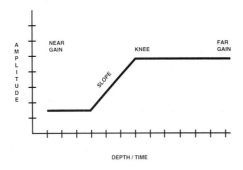

Figure 1-8. Time gain compensation curve.

52. 1. E, 2. A, 3. C, 4. F, 5. B, 6. D (See Fig. 1-8.)[1-6]

53. D. The sound velocity in the soft tissues of the body falls into a fairly small range, generally 1480 to 1640 m/s at normal body temperature. Therefore, an average velocity of 1540 m/s is used in most imaging systems.[5]

54. C. Modern ultrasound systems are calibrated to measure echo return time and calculate distance from the transducer face to the anatomic structure producing the echo. This distance is calculated using the following formula:

$$\text{distance to reflector} = \frac{\text{round trip time (s)} \times \text{velocity (cm/s)}}{2} \quad [5]$$

55. A. It is the amount of acoustic impedance mismatch that determines the percentage of sound reflected from an interface of a particular size. Echo amplitude is dependent on an acoustic impedance mismatch that increases the acoustic impedance differences between the two media, thereby increasing the amplitude of the returning echo.[4]

56. D. Spatial pulse length (SPL) is the length of the pulse in space and is equal to the wavelength of the center frequency multiplied by the number of cycles in the pulse. Axial resolution is dependent on SPL because it is equal to one-half the SPL (i.e., able to resolve two interfaces as separate interfaces if the distance between them is equal to or greater than one-half the SPL).[4]

57. B. Normally, TGC delay is not used in abdominal scanning. It is used, however, to delay the start of the TGC curve and is helpful when some sort of material layer with an unusual attenuation rate exists between the transducer and the organs being imaged. A thick layer of subcutaneous fat should be handled with a delay through the fat layer, after which the TGC ramp would be started into the organs.[14]

58. D. Cavitation may be either stable or transient. With stable cavitation, resonating microbubbles produce a violent disturbance in surrounding tissue, which also may give rise to microstreaming capable of causing shear stresses in molecules and cells and resulting in damage. This cavitation is not shown to occur with the short pulse duration that exists with diagnostic instrumentation. Transient cavitation produces shock waves during the compression phase of the cycle. In addition, high temperatures and pressures that occur within the bubbles are responsible for the decomposition of water into free radicals; this has never been shown to occur in tissue.[4]

59. A. One of the limitations of color-flow Doppler is the artifactual appearance of a color different from those which correctly represent normal forward/reverse flow. This is known as the *aliasing artifact.*[6]

60. C. In order to generate sound, something mechanical must move in a to-and-fro motion. In ultrasound, a piezoelectric transducer serves as a mechanical device pushing out during the first half of the cycle. Molecules immediately adjacent to it are compressed. During the second half of the cycle, the device moves back to its original position, causing those molecules to become less compressed, or rarefied. An entire cycle, then, consists of a compression phase and a rarefaction phase.[2, 10]

61. B. Pioneering sonographers scanned patients in immersion tanks filled with water or saline solutions. These liquids were chosen because they were plentiful, cheap, and had an impedance of 1.48, which compares nicely with the acoustic impedance of soft tissue,

which is approximately 1.63. With developing technology, mineral and castor oil (acoustic impedance of 1.43) replaced water as a coupling agent for early contact scanning. The emergence of real-time transducers introduced a clear, aqueous gel (with an impedance approximately the same as water) as the coupling agent of choice for all real-time scanning.[2]

62. B. The *Q factor*, or quality factor, of a transducer is equal to the resonant frequency divided by the bandwidth; high-Q transducers tend to ring for a long time, while low-Q transducers tend to ring for a shorter period and yield better resolution.[16]

63. D. In diagnostic ultrasound one is interested in comparing intensities. Two intensities may be compared by calculating the ratio of one to the other. Since sonographers encounter very wide ranges of such ratios, a linear scale would be very awkward. Therefore, a more manageable, logarithmic scale has been adopted. This decibel scale has many convenient attributes: It permits comparison of a wide number of intensity ratios, it is additive or subtractive when intensities are multiplied or subdivided, and it permits the use of negative decibel values to represent attenuation or reduction of intensity.[6, 10]

64. A. Bandwidth is the range of frequencies, or difference between the highest and the lowest frequencies emitted by a transducer. A transducer that emits only a few other frequencies on either side of the main frequency is called a *narrow-bandwidth transducer*. Transducers that emit many frequencies on either side of the main frequency are considered to have a wide bandwidth. Since bandwidth influences the imaging characteristics of transducers, wide bandwidths are preferable.[6, 16]

65. A. The fraction of the beam that encounters an interface determines the amount of energy reflected. Specular interfaces are large and smooth with respect to the wavelength of the sound beam, and will reflect a great deal of sound.[5]

66. C. The duty factor is equal to the pulse duration divided by the pulse repetition period (PRP).[4, 6, 14]

67. A. The annular-array transducer consists of a round crystal cut into concentric rings. By firing the rings in rapid sequence, the effective beam is concentrated in the center.[5]

68. C. An ultrasound wave is said to suffer absorption as it propagates.

The mechanical energy extracted from the wave by absorption mechanisms is converted into heat in the medium.[4-10]

69. C. Propagation speed is a property of the media. If you know the frequency, you can find the wavelength, or vice versa.

$$V = fx/\text{wavelength}$$

To solve this problem, the wavelength is calculated by dividing the velocity (1540 m/s) by the frequency (3.5 MHz).[1-6]

70. E

71. A

72. B

73. D

74. C[1-6]

75. B. The formula for computing acoustic impedance is expressed as:

$$Z = cp$$

Z = acoustic impedance (rayls), p = density (g/cm^3), and c = velocity of sound (cm/s). A rayl is a unit of measure of impedance (1 rayl = 1 kg/m^2/s).[16]

76. C. A ghost artifact is one in which the beam is refracted by the rectus muscles, thereby causing doubling or tripling of the initial (true) reflection. A ghost artifact, like all true artifacts, can be produced in only one scan plane, so rotating the transducer 90° and rescanning the same area will cause a reduction in the number of duplicated objects (echoes).[3]

77. C[11]

78. D

79. E

80. B

81. A

82. C[1-6]

83. D. The highest-frequency transducer that allows adequate penetration should be used. The superficially located thyroid gland must fall within the focal range of the transducer. Typically, this is a 7.5 or 10 MHz with a short focal length. If the thyroid lesion is deep within the neck, a medium focal length would provide the necessary penetration and acceptable resolution.[2, 16]

84. C. With pulse-echo equipment, the crystal vibrates for a relatively short time and "listens" for a relatively long time. In general, the crystal pulses 1% of the time and receives the remaining 99%.[2]

85. D. A large percentage of routine sonography involves the recognition, use, or elimination of artifacts. For instance, gallstones produce a shadowing artifact that is essential to diagnosis. Artifacts that confuse or obscure an image can be eliminated in some cases by avoiding beam perpendicularity to strong interfaces. However, some artifacts are related to the physical properties of the transmitting medium; they cannot be used or eliminated and must be recognized and reported as artifacts.[1-6]

86. D. In addition to the traditional wire and pin phantoms, there are tissue-mimicking (TM) phantoms specifically designed to exhibit the acoustic parameters of soft tissue. In addition, they contain structures—nylon wires and "cysts" of different diameters, high-amplitude scattering lesions, and simulated vessels. All these materials are sensitive to the various imaging parameters and can be used to obtain measurements of beamwidth, focal zone, near and far zones, and scanner electronic circuit malfunctions.[7]

87. C. Side lobe artifacts are caused by the presence of multiple, lower-intensity sound beams located outside the main beam. At most, they are $1/100$ the intensity of the main beam (20 dB or lower). Side lobe artifacts may be either diffuse or specular in appearance and occur when sufficiently intense transducer side lobes interact with highly reflective acoustic surfaces. Specular side lobe artifacts are associated with curved, highly reflecting surfaces such as the diaphragm, urinary bladder, or gallbladder. Diffuse side lobe artifact echoes are most apparent when highly reflective bowel gas lies adjacent to a cystic organ. Because side lobe echoes are much less intense than those originating within the main beam, they exhibit a threshold effect and will disappear with lower instrument settings, whereas real echoes will persist. Side lobes are angle-dependent; therefore, a change in transducer angulation and/or repositioning

the transducer away from gas-filled or highly reflective structures should diminish or eliminate these troublesome echoes.[12]

88. B. Annular phased-array scanners combine the best features of both mechanical and linear-array scanners. Because the computer-fired elements are aligned concentrically, instead of in a row, a narrow cylindrical beam can be created. Annular-array beams have a high signal-to-noise ratio over a wide focal zone and permit the use of higher-frequency transducers. The transmit beam is electronically regulated so that transmit focus can be user-selected for the appropriate depth. Electronic phasing also permits dynamic receive-focusing that is independent of transmit-focus, thus ensuring optimal tissue clarity throughout the depth of field. Beam penetration is good in fatty patients because the annular array lacks the tremendous side lobes and scattering problems often seen with linear phased arrays.[4–6]

89. C

90. E

91. D

92. B

93. A[4, 6, 9]

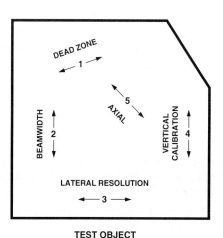

Figure 1-9. AIUM standard 100-mm test object.

94. 1. D, 2. A, 3. E, 4. C, 5. B (See Fig. 1-9.)[7]

95. C. Energy output controls affect the amount of energy leaving a transducer and operate by varying the excitation voltage or the amount of transducer damping. Amplification of echoes is a receiver function.[13]

96. C (0.000001)

97. D (0.001)

98. E (0.01)

99. A (1,000)

100. B (1,000,000)[6]

101. D. It was the scan converter that made gray scale possible by storing the image and then displaying it on a CRT. Images can be manipulated or altered between storage and display of the data. At first, analog scan converters were used, but problems of image flickering, fading, drifting, and deterioration made them unacceptable. Digital scan converters were then adopted, primarily because they utilized computer memory to digitize images. By converting the image into numbers and storing the numbers in memory, it was possible to process or manipulate them and then retranslate and display them as an image. Digital scan converters are more stable and do not suffer from the problems inherent in analog scan converters.[6,9]

102. B. Output power controls are provided on some instruments, allowing the sonographer to vary the sensitivity of the ultrasound system. If the output power to the transducer is increased, higher-intensity transmit pulses and larger-amplitude signals result to allow visualization of weaker echoes.[6,9,14]

103. B. Preprocessing allows manipulation of the digital data *before* it is stored in the scan converter but *after* it is in digital format.[6]

104. D. Among the important features of a spectrum are how long it appears, what direction blood is flowing, and what maximum and mean velocities can be demonstrated. *Spectral broadening* refers to the range of frequencies present. Excessive instrument gain or blood turbulence creates ambiguity.[6,11] (Courtesy of Lynda Ranson, Orange Coast College, Costa Mesa, California.)

105. B. Imaging with a single pulse to a specific depth requires time, as

does creating a single frame with a large number of pulses and presenting many frames in rapid sequence. Therefore, imaging depth, lines per frame, and frame rate duel for time. A compromise must be made to balance these factors.[9] (Courtesy of Marsha Wolfson, Orange Coast College, Costa Mesa, California.)

106. C. Shadowing is the reduction in the reflection amplitude from the reflectors that lie behind a strongly reflecting or attenuating structure.[9]

107. B. Sources of beam deflection include refraction and reflections at specular interfaces. Since the displayed echo position is along the line of sight of the transducer beam axis, echo signals could appear on a B-scan image in a position quite remote from their actual anatomic origin.[9]

108. C. Cavitation is the production of microbubbles. It occurs when dissolved gases grow into bubbles around stable microbubble nuclei during the negative-pressure phase of the propagated sound wave.[2]

109. C. In a mirror-image artifact, objects that are present on one side of a strong reflector are represented on the other side as well.[11]

110. D. All except the mirror image depend in some way on characteristics of the pulse.[6]

111. B. A mirror-image artifact occurs when a pulse bounces off a strong reflector (such as the diaphragm) and then strikes a second reflector. The path of the pulse is lengthened by the mirroring, and the second reflection is always displayed at an abnormally greater depth.[6] (Courtesy of James Pennington, Johns Hopkins School of Ultrasound, Baltimore, Maryland.)

112. D. A-mode (amplitude modulation) is diagnostic ultrasound information displayed as the amplitude of an electrical signal along a baseline. The stronger the reflecting surface, the higher in amplitude is the returning echo. The time line (distance line) is calibrated in centimeters. In an A-mode tracing, solid structures will produce a cluster of variable echo amplitudes. The absence of echoes indicates that the medium is homogeneous and contains no internal echo-reflecting interfaces.[2, 4, 14]

113. C. Brightness modulation (B-mode) information is applied to the Z axis of the oscilloscope instead of the vertical deflection circuit. Echoes appear as intensified points of illumination along a base

line. B-mode is not useful in itself but is used to create M-mode (motion-mode) and B-scan displays.[6, 11, 14]

114. C. An acoustic window is an area through which the sound beam can pass unimpeded. First, the sonographer must avoid transducer-air-tissue interfaces at the skin surface. Once an air-free contact between the transducer and skin is achieved, the sonographer is ready to search for an acoustic window. Fluid-filled structures, such as the stomach, urinary bladder, and gallbladder, are among the best acoustic windows.[16]

115. F

116. A

117. C

118. E

119. D

120. B[2, 6, 11]

121. B. One of the most popular man-made crystals is lead zirconate titanate, or PZT.[6, 11]

REFERENCES

1. Athey PA, McClendon L. Diagnostic ultrasound for radiographers. Denver: Multi-Media Publishing, 1983.

2. Bushong SC, Archer BR. Ultrasound physics, biology, and instrumentation. St. Louis: Mosby-Year Book, 1991.

3. Buttery B, Davison G. The ghost artifact. J Ultrasound Med 1984; 3:49.

4. Buurma G, Fuller DC, Goddard J. Guidelines for physics review. 3rd ed. Dallas: Society of Diagnostic Medical Sonographers, 1992.

5. Craig M. Diagnostic medical sonography. Vol 2: Echocardiography. Philadelphia: JB Lippincott, 1991.

6. Edelman SK. Understanding ultrasound physics. Houston: ESP Publishers, 1990.

7. Goldstein, A. Quality assurance in diagnostic ultrasound: a quality assurance manual for the clinical user. Bethesda: American Institute of Ultrasound in Medicine, 1980.

8. Goldstein A. Ultrasound devices open new diagnostic avenues. Diagnostic Imaging, Sept. 1989; 157.

9. Hagen-Ansert SL. Textbook of diagnostic sonography. 3rd ed. St. Louis: CV Mosby, 1989.

10. Hussey M. Basic physics and technology of medical diagnostic ultrasound. London: Macmillan, 1985.

11. Kremkau FW. Diagnostic ultrasound: principles, instruments, and exercises. Philadelphia: WB Saunders, 1989.

12. Laing FC. Commonly encountered artifacts in clinical ultrasound. Sem Ultrasound 1983; 4(1):27.

13. Pinkney N. A review of the concepts of ultrasound physics and instrumentation. West Point, PA: Sonicor, 1983.

14. Powis R, Powis WJ. A thinker's guide to ultrasonic imaging. Baltimore: Urban & Swarzenberg, 1984.

15. Sanders RC. Clinical sonography, a practical guide. 2nd ed. Boston: Little Brown, 1991.

16. Wicks JD, Howe KS. Fundamentals of ultrasonographic technique. Chicago: Year Book Medical Publishers, 1983.

Marveen Craig: *Ultrasound Exam Review*, © 1994 J. B. Lippincott Co.

2

Abdomen

OBJECTIVES

Of all of the clinical applications of diagnostic ultrasound, abdominal sonography encompasses the greatest range of major organs and systems. The corresponding array of congenital anomalies and potential pathologies is staggering. Therefore, the abdominal sonographer is challenged to develop extensive knowledge of the anatomy, physiology, and sonographic appearance of each of the abdominal organs as well as the myriad changes introduced by disease. With that in mind, this chapter emphasizes anatomy and physiology, as well as concentrating on the pathologies most commonly encountered in modern ultrasound settings.

QUESTIONS

Directions

Each of the questions or incomplete statements is followed by several answers or completions. Select the best answer(s) in each case. In the matching sections, answers should be used only once, unless otherwise stated.

1. The clinical triad of elevated temperature, leukocytosis, and swelling or tenderness are symptomatic of:
   A. developing hematoma.
   B. inflammatory process.
   C. malignant neoplasm.
   D. all of the above

2. Which of the following will adversely affect a sonographic study of the abdomen?
   A. Ileus and dehydration
   B. Bowel gas
   C. Barium and endoscopic studies
   D. All of the above

3. Hemangiomas can be differentiated into two types:
   A. ductal and strophal.
   B. capillary and ductal.
   C. cavernous and capillary.
   D. cavernous and strophal.

4. The sonographic features of advanced cirrhosis include all of the following except:
   A. splenomegaly.
   B. portal vein aneurysm.
   C. recanalized umbilical vein.
   D. varices.

5. The progression of autosomal dominant polycystic kidney disease may show cystic changes in other organs. Which of the following is not a site for concomitant polycystic changes?
   A. Pancreas
   B. Adrenals
   C. Liver
   D. Testes

6. Identify the numbered structures in Figure 2-1.

   1. ___   A. Minor calyx
   2. ___   B. Renal pelvis
   3. ___   C. Renal medulla
                    (pyramids)
   4. ___   D. Renal artery
   5. ___   E. Papilla
   6. ___   F. Major calyx
   7. ___   G. Renal vein
   8. ___   H. Cortex

7. Biliary cirrhosis may be caused by all of the following entities except:
   A. alcohol abuse.

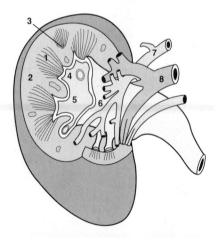

Figure 2-1. Illustration of the kidney in cross-section.

B. chronic viral hepatitis.
C. jaundice.
D. Wilson's disease.

8. Which of the following statements regarding retroperitoneal fibrosis is *untrue*?
   A. Generally confined to the para-vertebral and central regions of the abdomen
   B. May be associated with bilateral ureteral obstruction
   C. Sonographic appearance of a hyperechoic midline mass
   D. May produce back pain, weight loss, and hypertension

9. The sandwich sign describes the ultrasonic depiction of:
   A. the pancreas draped over the prevertebral vessels.
   B. nodes lying anterior and posterior to the SMA.
   C. nodes surrounding and flattening the celiac axis.
   D. the relationship of the cystic duct, hepatic artery, and the portal vein.

10. The dividing point between the right and left liver lobes is the:
    A. main lobar fissure.
    B. ligamentum teres.
    C. ligamentum venosum.
    D. falciform ligament.

11. Segmental division of the liver is clinically important when surgical resection is being considered. Sonographers can define the two right and two left segments and the caudate lobe by the primary branching of the:
    A. portal vein.

B. hepatic artery.
C. hepatic veins.
D. A and B

12. The transducer of choice for examining the average-sized, normal adult liver is a:
    A. 2 MHz.
    B. 3.5 MHz.
    C. 5 MHz.
    D. 7.5 MHz.

13. Which of the following statements is *not* a characteristic of a horseshoe kidney?
    A. May present as a pulsatile abdominal mass
    B. Majority are fused at upper poles
    C. Generally asymptomatic
    D. Usually located at iliac crest

14. Laboratory test(s) that may be elevated with hepatic metastatic disease include:
    A. amylase and lipase.
    B. alpha-fetoprotein.
    C. carcino-embryonic antigen.
    D. B and C

15. Identify the numbered structures in Figure 2-2.

1. ___	A. Pancreas
2. ___	B. Spleen
3. ___	C. Inferior mesenteric vein
4. ___	D. Liver
5. ___	E. Inferior pancreaticoduodenal vein
6. ___	F. Left portal vein
7. ___	G. Left gastro-epiploic vein
8. ___	H. Right colic vein

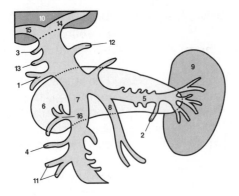

Figure 2-2. Illustration of portal vein formation.

9. ___   I. Right gastro-
            epiploic vein
10. ___   J. Right portal
            vein
11. ___   K. Splenic vein
12. ___   L. Superior mes-
            enteric vein
13. ___   M. Superior pan-
            creaticoduode-
            nal vein
14. ___   N. Accessory pan-
            creatic vein
15. ___   O. Cystic vein
16. ___   P. Right gastric
            vein (pyloric)

16. The presence of a hetero-
    geneous thickening of the gall-
    bladder wall, pericholecystic
    fluid collections, and intra-
    luminal membranes are so-
    nographic signs of:
    A. a ruptured gallbladder.
    B. a porcelain gallbladder.
    C. a Courvoisier gallbladder.
    D. gangrenous cholecystitis.

17. Hodgkin's disease is a malig-
    nant condition characterized
    by painless, progressive en-
    largement of the lymph nodes,
    spleen, and general lymphoid
    tissue. Which of the following
    are characteristic of Hodgkin's
    disease?
    A. Weight loss, night sweats,
       intermittent fever, pruritis
    B. Multiple hypoechoic or hy-
       perechoic masses
    C. Complicated by the develop-
       ment of hemolytic anemia
    D. Inflammatory changes are
       an intrinsic component

18. The tongue-like projection of
    tissue that extends between
    the inferior vena cava (IVC)
    and portal vein (PV) is the:
    A. caudate lobe.
    B. quadrate lobe.
    C. caudate process.
    D. quadrate process.

19. Resolution of adrenal hemor-
    rhage is sometimes followed by
    the development of:
    A. calcifications.
    B. cysts.
    C. capsular thickening.
    D. adrenal agenesis.

20. Compared to hepatic veins, the
    portal veins can be distin-
    guished by their sonographic
    pattern of:
    A. high-amplitude wall echoes.
    B. low-amplitude wall echoes.
    C. drainage into the inferior
       vena cava.
    D. gallbladder proximity.

21. Which of the following anatom-
    ical landmarks are commonly

used to identify the neck of the gallbladder?
A. Right portal vein, main lobar fissure
B. Main portal vein, cystic duct
C. Hepatic artery, common bile duct
D. Ligamentum venosum, valves of Heister

22. Non-Hodgkin's lymphomas are solid tumors arising in the peripheral lympho-reticular tissues (particularly those of the lymph nodes), the oro-pharynx, the gut, skin, and other sites. Which of the following comments about non-Hodgkin's lymphomas is (are) true?
A. Epstein-Barr virus infection may cause Burkitt's lymphoma
B. May show evidence of ecotaxis
C. Tumors arising in lymph nodes spread only to other nodes
D. Enlarged cervical nodes are seen with mononucleosis

23. Which of the following are pitfalls in adrenal sonography?
A. Esophagogastric junction mimicking the left adrenal
B. Crus of the diaphragm may be mistaken for adrenal pathology; fatty tumors may cause diaphragmatic echo disruption
C. Adrenal gland easily mistaken for kidney in cases of renal agenesis
D. All of the above

24. One of the liver's functions is to produce bilirubin from old red blood cells. The bilirubin laboratory test results can be read as direct increases or indirect increases. An increase in the direct (conjugated) bilirubin signifies _____, whereas an increase in the indirect (unconjugated) bilirubin signifies _____.
A. obstruction; hepatocellular disease
B. jaundice; polycythemia
C. hepatocellular disease; obstruction
D. polycythemia; jaundice

25. The term *portal triad* describes the arrangement of the following structures within the hepatocytes:
A. hepatic artery, hepatic vein, biliary radicle.
B. hepatic artery, portal vein, bile duct.
C. inferior mesenteric vein, portal vein, hepatic vein.
D. portal venule, hepatic arteriole, biliary sinusoid.

26. Which of the following statements concerning renal transplantation is (are) *not true*?
A. Requires use of highest frequency transducer available
B. Psoas muscle lies posterior to transplanted kidney
C. Immunologic rejection produces edema
D. Distinct corticomedullary boundaries appear with acute rejection

27. Identify the vessels of the upper abdomen shown in Figure 2-3.

    1. ___   A. Lumbar artery
    2. ___   B. Celiac trunk
    3. ___   C. Renal Vein
    4. ___   D. Hepatic artery
    5. ___   E. External iliac arteries
    6. ___   F. Suprarenal (adrenal) artery
    7. ___   G. Left gastric artery
    8. ___   H. Abdominal aorta
    9. ___   I. Internal iliac arteries
    10. ___   J. Testicular/ovarian arteries
    11. ___   K. Middle sacral artery
    12. ___   L. Splenic artery
    13. ___   M. Inferior mesenteric artery
    14. ___   N. Common iliac arteries
    15. ___   O. Superior mesenteric artery
    16. ___   P. Inferior phrenic artery

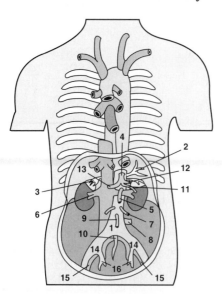

Figure 2-3. Abdominal aorta and tributaries.

28. Which of the following laboratory test findings is *not* associated with acute pancreatitis?
    A. Elevated fasting blood sugars (FBS)
    B. Elevated serum bilirubin and liver enzymes
    C. Elevated serum amylase
    D. Elevated leukocytes and AFP

29. Early in the formation of ascites, minimal fluid collections can usually be found in the:
    A. subphrenic space.
    B. Retzian space.
    C. subhepatic space.
    D. perinephric space.

30. The medial segment of the left lobe of the liver was formerly known as the:
    A. caudate lobe.
    B. Reidel's lobe.
    C. quadrate lobe.
    D. Morrison's lobe

31. Pseudohydronephrosis occurs as a result of:
    A. the presence of renal calculi.
    B. prolonged prostatic enlargement.
    C. an overly distended bladder.
    D. patient obesity.

32. The *mantle effect* is an ultrasound term coined to describe:

A. enlarged intrahepatic ducts.
B. para-aortic lymphadenopathy.
C. a specific reverberation artifact.
D. configuration of the SM parallelling the aorta.

33. The thickness of the gallbladder wall in normal, preprandial patients is _____, while gallbladder wall thickness in postprandial patients is _____.
A. 2 mm; 4 mm
B. 3 mm; 5 mm
C. 4 mm; 3 mm
D. 3 mm; 3 mm

34. Laboratory evaluation of liver function can be achieved with a variety of tests. Which of the following tests shows a decrease in the presence of hepatocellular disease?
A. Bilirubin
B. Prothrombin time
C. Fetal antigen
D. Alkaline phosphatase

35. Hematuria is an important indicator of genitourinary problems. Which of the following conditions is *not* associated with hematuria?
A. Tumors or calculi
B. Prostatic hypertrophy
C. Diverticula
D. Perivesical hematoma

36. The liver receives its dual blood supply from the:
A. hepatic vein and portal vein.
B. portal vein and superior mesenteric artery.

C. superior mesenteric vein and hepatic artery.
D. portal vein and hepatic artery.

37. Polycystic kidney disease (PKD) is transmitted as either an autosomal dominant, or autosomal recessive, genetic disorder. The dominant form is also known as _____, while the recessive form is also known as _____.
A. multicystic dysplastic kidney disease; glomerulonephritis
B. infantile polycystic kidney disease; Potter's disease
C. tubular ectasia; nephrocalcinosis
D. adult PKD; infantile PKD

38. Which of the following entities are commonly associated with the spleen?
A. Accessory spleens
B. Cavernous hemangiomas
C. Lymphomas
D. A and C

39. The sonographic demonstration of microbubbles within an abscess is indicative of:
A. calcific formation.
B. gas formation.
C. stasis.
D. hematoma.

40. A 2-year-old female was scheduled for abdominal sonography because of increasing abdominal girth despite a failure to thrive. Sonography revealed the presence of a large, heterogeneous mass displacing the

right kidney and crossing the midline. The mass also showed evidence of internal calcifications. Such findings most likely represent a:

A. nephroblastoma.
B. angiomyolipoma.
C. neuroblastoma.
D. pheochromocytoma.

41. Which of the following statements is *uncharacteristic* of the prostate gland?

A. It is a retroperitoneal structure.
B. It consists of four lobes.
C. It lies caudal to the seminal vesicles.
D. It is divided into internal and peripheral external zones.

42. The sonographic appearance of acute hepatitis differs from chronic hepatitis in that with acute forms of hepatitis, the liver becomes _____, whereas in chronic forms of hepatitis the liver becomes _____.

A. hyperechoic; hypoechoic
B. isoechoic; hypoechoic
C. hypoechoic; hyperechoic
D. hyperechoic; isoechoic

43. Increased echogenicity of the pancreas is associated with:

A. suppurating pancreatitis.
B. cystic fibrosis.
C. chronic pancreatitis.
D. B and C

44. The proper technique for sonographic measurement of ducts is:

A. the leading edge technique.

B. internal wall diameters.
C. external wall diameters.
D. B and C

45. Identify the structures in Figure 2-4.

1. ___   A. Inferior vena cava
2. ___   B. Bare area
3. ___   C. Right lobe
4. ___   D. Gallbladder
5. ___   E. Medial segment of left lobe
6. ___   F. Cystic duct
7. ___   G. Hepatic duct
8. ___   H. Portal vein
9. ___   I. Ligamentum teres
10. ___   J. Caudate lobe
11. ___   K. Left lobe
12. ___   L. Falciform ligament

46. Structures that may mimic stones in the common duct include all of the following *except:*

A. gas in the duodenum.
B. biliary air or post-

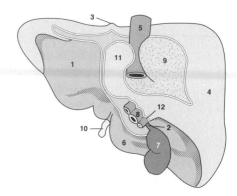

Figure 2-4. Posterior view of the diaphragmatic surface of the liver.

cholecystectomy surgical
clips.

C. fluid in the duodenum.

D. calcifications in the head of
the pancreas.

47. In some patients with fatty in-
filtrative or cirrhotic disease,
the _____ lobe is often the site
of focal sparing.
A. caudate
B. Reidel's
C. left
D. medial segment of left lobe

48. In scanning patients with
known acute trauma, the sonographer must also look for
evidence of:
A. the butterfly sign.
B. Morrison's pouch.
C. fluid in the lesser sac and
greater sac.
D. all of the above

49. Sonography can provide excellent measurements of the extrahepatic bile ducts. The
upper limits of normal size of
the common hepatic duct
(CHD) and the common bile
duct (CBD) are:
A. 2–4 mm; 5–7 mm
B. 0.5 cm; 1 cm
C. 4–5 mm; 6–8 mm
D. 3 mm; 7 mm

50. The sonographic pattern of a
discrete round/oval abnormality with dense central echoes
and an anechoic periphery is a
sign of stomach or bowel abnormalities. Such lesions are
frequently called a:
A. doughnut sign.

B. target or bull's-eye sign.

C. tip of the iceberg sign.

D. halo sign.

51. In patients who have had a re-
cent oral cholecystogram, so-
nography of the gallbladder
may demonstrate:
A. "ringdown" artifacts.
B. "artificial" enhancement.
C. "sedentary" sludge.
D. "floating" stones.

52. Which of the following statements about the hepatic veins
is *untrue?*
A. Contain minimal amounts
of collagen
B. Demonstrate weak wall
echoes
C. Expand during Valsalva's
maneuver
D. Vessel diameter increases
near the porta hepatis

53. Hepatic abnormalities are common in acquired immunodefi-
ciency syndrome (AIDS) and
usually secondary to oppor-
tunistic infections or drugs.
The most common hepatic
neoplasm in AIDS is:
A. non-Hodgkin's lymphoma.
B. hemangioma.
C. Kaposi's sarcoma.
D. cholangioma.

54. The sonographic appearance of
(1) an impacted stone in the
cystic duct or neck of the gallbladder, (2) dilated biliary
ducts proximal to the calculus,
and (3) a normal-sized common bile duct distal to the cal-

culus describes the following syndrome:
A. Mirizzi.
B. Courvoisier.
C. Bouveret.
D. Rokitansky.

55. The parenchyma of the kidney is comprised of:
A. the tubule and corpuscles.
B. glomeruli and nephrons.
C. the cortex and renal pyramids.
D. Bowman's capsule and loops of Henle.

56. Which statement concerning congenital hepatic cysts is false?
A. Are developmental defects of bile ducts
B. Are asymptomatic and rarely cause hepatomegaly or jaundice
C. Are more often solitary than multiple
D. Left-lobe incidence is greater than right lobe

57. The WES triad relates to examination of patients with contracted or nonvisualized gallbladders. The acronym "WES" refers to:
A. "wide-echo-shadow."
B. "wall-echolucent-stone."
C. "wall-echo-shadow."
D. "wall-edema-sludge."

58. The presence of calcifications within liver metastases is suggestive of a mucinous adenocarcinoma as the primary neoplasm. The most common

location(s) for this type of mass is (are) the:
A. pancreas and kidneys.
B. colon.
C. ovaries.
D. B and C

59. In the presence of splenomegaly, the sonographer should also examine the:
A. lymphatic system.
B. the liver.
C. the portal system.
D. all of the above

60. The echogenicity of the pancreas should be compared to the liver. A normal pancreas should demonstrate an echogenicity that is _____ or _____ the liver:
A. equal to; less than
B. equal to; greater than
C. less than; greater than
D. greater than; less than

61. Simple renal cyst is associated with all of the following findings *except:*
A. an increased incidence in older age groups.
B. that it is uncommon in infants and children.
C. gross hematuria.
D. partial obstruction of the collecting system.

62. Which of the following statements about advanced cirrhosis of the liver is *false?*
A. Associated with increased echogenicity and attenuation
B. Associated with hepatosplenomegaly

C. Associated with recanalization of the umbilical vein
D. Associated with liver parenchyma appearing less echogenic than renal parenchyma

63. The duct of Wirsung is considered abnormal if the lumen is greater than:
    A. 1 mm.
    B. 2 mm.
    C. 3 mm.
    D. 4 mm.

64. Disease of the kidney associated with increased cortical echogenicity include(s):
    A. acute, chronic glomerulonephritis.
    B. diffuse infiltrating lymphoma.
    C. infantile polycystic kidney disease.
    D. all of the above

65. Which of the following statements about sludge is *untrue*?
    A. Usually occupies the dependent portion of the gallbladder
    B. Produces acoustic "shadowing"
    C. May clump together (tumefaction) to form masses or balls
    D. Considered a precursor to biliary disease

66. Compared to the liver, the most echogenic portion of the kidneys is (are) the _____. The least echogenic portion of the kidney is the _____.
    A. renal sinuses and peri-renal fat; renal pyramids

B. renal cortex; renal capsule
C. renal medulla; renal cortex
D. renal capsule; medullary junction

67. Echogenic bile is often found in patients with extrahepatic biliary obstruction and acute and chronic cholecystitis, as well as in patients undergoing fasts or hyperalimentation. Biliary stasis, the common denominator in these cases, will produce sludge. The composition of sludge is mainly:
    A. hematobilia.
    B. calcium bilirubinate crystals.
    C. calcium phosphatase.
    D. cholesterolosis.

68. The term *porcelain gallbladder* refers to:
    A. milk of calcium within the gallbladder.
    B. empyema of the gallbladder.
    C. hyperechoic mural foci.
    D. residual barium within the gallbladder.

69. With hepatocellular carcinoma, Doppler signals and the resistive index of the tumor vessels are _____ as the vessels progress into the center of the lesion.
    A. increased
    B. decreased
    C. identical
    D. absent

70. Which of the following statements apply to the left renal vein?
    A. Runs anterior to the supe-

rior mesenteric artery (SMA)
B. Is shorter than the right renal vein
C. Runs anterior to abdominal aorta and inferior vena cava
D. A and D

71. Comparing the caudate lobe to right lobe size is valuable in diagnosing the presence of cirrhosis. When ratios are _____, cirrhosis is indicated:
A. greater than 45–50%
B. greater than 55–60%
C. greater than 65–70%
D. less than 60%

72. Which of the following conditions does *not* produce jaundice?
A. Adenomyomatosis of the gallbladder
B. Klatskin tumor
C. Courvoisier gallbladder
D. Hepatitis

73. Successful pancreatography requires detailed understanding of the surrounding vasculature. Blood supply to the pancreas is provided by branches of the:
A. splenic, vagal, and mesenteric arteries.
B. splenic vein and artery and superior mesenteric vein and artery.
C. gastroduodenal, splenic, and superior mesenteric arteries.
D. celiac, inferior mesenteric, and portal vessels.

74. The sonographic features of advanced cirrhosis include all of the following *except:*
A. splenomegaly.
B. portal vein aneurysm.
C. recanalized umbilical vein.
D. varices.

75. The Budd-Chiari syndrome refers to:
A. congenital abnormality of the biliary system.
B. congenitally anomalous left liver lobe.
C. hepatic venous outflow obstruction.
D. hepatic artery atresia.

76. Which of the following statements about metastatic gallbladder disease is *untrue?*
A. Metastases from malignant melanoma is most common
B. May mimic acute or chronic cholecystitis
C. Associated with gallstones
D. Not as rare as once thought

77. Which of the following conditions do patients on chronic hemodialysis often develop?
A. Multiple small renal cysts
B. Renal neoplasms
C. Lymphoceles and urinomas
D. A and B

78. A dramatically enlarged gallbladder filled with clear mucous is referred to as a:
A. mucocele and hydropic gallbladder.
B. hydrocele.
C. porcelain gallbladder.
D. A and C

79. Parenchymal cysts that bulge into the central sinus of the kidney are known as _____, whereas _____ are lymphatic cysts in the central sinus of the kidney.
    A. peri-pelvic; extra-paren-chymal
    B. para-pelvic; medullary
    C. para-pelvic; peri-pelvic
    D. peri-pelvic; cortical

80. Which of the following conditions is *not* associated with splenomegaly?
    A. Collagen diseases
    B. Malaria
    C. Sickle-cell anemia
    D. Chronic granulocytic leukemia

81. Downward displacement of the superior mesenteric artery (SMA) is associated with:
    A. pseudocyst formation.
    B. pancreatitis.
    C. pancreatic neoplasm.
    D. acute cholecystitis.

82. Thickening of the gallbladder wall is seen in all of the following *except:*
    A. acute cholecystitis.
    B. hydrops.
    C. contracted gallbladder.
    D. ascites.

83. Which of the following statements regarding color Doppler and pulsed wave Doppler examination of the spleen is (are) true?
    A. Splenic vein blood flow is continuous, of low velocity, and is similar to portal vein blood flow.
    B. Splenic artery flow peaks in systole and declines in diastole.
    C. Blood flow is easily demonstrated at the splenic hilus.
    D. All of the above

84. Extension of renal carcinoma into the inferior vena cava occurs through the:
    A. lymph nodes.
    B. portal vein.
    C. renal vein.
    D. renal artery.

85. Abdominal sonography was ordered on a 23-year-old black male with a history of exposure to hepatitis but without history of alcohol or intravenous drug abuse. Blood studies were positive for hepatitis-B; SGOT, SGPT, alkaline phosphatase, and bilirubin were elevated. Serum alpha-fetoprotein was markedly elevated. Sonography revealed hepatomegaly with marked enlargement of the left lobe. Irregular areas of increased echogenicity were seen in the left lobe, and a large focal area of densely increased echogenicity occupied the right lobe. Examination of the vascular system revealed a large solid mass within the portal veins. The most likely pathology in this patient is:
    A. hemangioma.
    B. hepatocellular carcinoma.
    C. regenerating cirrhotic nodule.
    D. A and C

86. A common gallbladder variant formed by the kinking or folding back of the fundus of the gallbladder onto its body is known as:
    A. Hartmann's pouch.
    B. Murphy's sign.
    C. Courvoisier's sign.
    D. a Phrygian cap.

87. Identify the structures shown in Figure 2-5.

1. ___	A. Common bile duct
2. ___	B. Cystic duct
3. ___	C. Cystic artery
4. ___	D. Common hepatic duct
5. ___	E. Proper hepatic artery
6. ___	F. Portal vein
7. ___	G. Common hepatic artery
8. ___	H. Pancreas
9. ___	I. Duodenum
10. ___	J. Gallbladder
11. ___	K. Liver
12. ___	L. Stomach

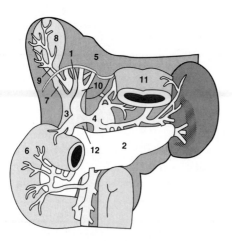

Figure 2-5. The biliary system.

88. Which of the following is *not* a test of renal function?
    A. BUN
    B. Cr cl
    C. UA
    D. AST

89. Of the following statements concerning pancreatic neoplasms, which is *untrue*?
    A. May mimic or be associated with acute pancreatitis
    B. Adenocarcinoma is the most common tumor
    C. Produces echogenicity greater than that of the liver
    D. Increased risk in smokers

90. Acute hepatitis produces sonographic changes in the echo pattern of portal veins. Compared with healthy patients, portal vein walls will appear:
    A. anechoic.
    B. isoechoic.
    C. hyperechoic.
    D. hypoechoic.

91. Pseudo-calculi may be demonstrated with sonography. The leading causes are:
    A. surgical clips.
    B. ductal air or gas.
    C. valves of Heister and adjacent bowel gas.
    D. all of the above

92. Following cholecystectomy, the common duct typically measures:
    A. 6 mm or less.
    B. less than 4 mm.
    C. 7 mm or more.
    D. up to 10 mm.

93. Abscesses that occupy the space between the liver and the diaphragm are known as _____ abscesses.
    A. subhepatic
    B. paracolic
    C. subphrenic
    D. intrahepatic

94. Pneumobilia is commonly associated with all of the following *except*:
    A. papillectomy.
    B. ERCP.
    C. Roux-en-Y procedures.
    D. sphincterotomy.

95. A patient with a positive Courvoisier's sign will exhibit:
    A. dilated and noncontracting gallbladder.
    B. epigastric mass or steatorrhea.
    C. epigastric pain radiating to the back.
    D. all of the above

96. Echinococcal cysts are associated with all of the following *except:*
    A. tapeworms.
    B. daughter cysts.
    C. calcification.
    D. aspiration techniques.

97. An increase in the size of the common duct (CD) is a sensitive indicator of biliary obstruction. The normal range of CD diameter in adult patients under 60 years of age is _____, whereas in patients over 60 the normal range is _____.
    A. 35 mm; 77 mm
    B. 5 mm; 6 mm

C. 3–4 mm; 5–6 mm
    D. 4–5 mm; 7–8 mm

98. Autodigestion of the pancreas occurs with:
    A. obstruction of the pancreatic ducts.
    B. pseudocyst formation.
    C. hepatosplenomegaly.
    D. A or B

99. Hepatomegaly is associated with:
    A. right heart failure.
    B. sonographic appearance of blunt liver edges.
    C. an increase of cells (intracellular or extracellular deposits).
    D. all of the above

100. Two of the more common malignant neoplasms of the pancreas are adenocarcinoma and cystadenocarcinoma. Adenocarcinomas arise primarily in the pancreatic _____. Cystadenocarcinomas are most often found in the _____.
    A. body and tail; head and body
    B. head; tail
    C. tail; head
    D. head and body; uncinate process

101. In a 40-year-old female patient complaining of hematuria and known tuberous sclerosis, the sonographic appearance of a highly echogenic, sound-attenuating unilateral mass is most suggestive of:
    A. hypernephroma.

B. mesoblastic nephroma.
C. angiomyolipoma.
D. pheochromocytoma.

102. Transcatheter arterial emboli-
     zation (TAE) is a therapeutic
     modality used for unresect-
     able hepatocellular car-
     cinoma. Doppler sonography
     may be a useful modality in
     the follow-up of response to
     TAE in patients with hepato-
     cellular carcinoma (HCC) be-
     cause it can demonstrate:
     A. detectable Doppler signals
        (within lesions after TAE),
        indicating patent tumor
        vessels.
     B. disappearance of detect-
        able Doppler signals after
        TAE, indicating that the
        patient is completely free
        of hepatocellular car-
        cinoma.
     C. increased velocity.
     D. decreased velocity.

103. Which of the following prepa-
     ration and scanning tech-
     niques are used to minimize
     the detrimental effects of
     bowel gas when performing
     abdominal sonography exam-
     inations?
     A. Use of methylcellulose
     B. Injection of glucagon
     C. Fasting or water ingestion
     D. All of the above

104. For evaluation of the right
     posterior lobe of the liver in
     an obese patient, the trans-
     ducer of choice would be:
     A. 5 MHz short focus.
     B. 7.5 MHz short focus.

C. 2.25 MHz deep focus.
D. 3.5 MHz medium focus.

105. Which of the following struc-
     tures can simulate the pan-
     creatic duct?
     A. Splenic artery or vein
     B. Posterior stomach wall
     C. Retroperitoneal fat
     D. All of the above

106. Which of the following is *not*
     an intrinsic cause of hydro-
     nephrosis?
     A. Calculous or clot
     B. Stricture
     C. Benign prostatic hypertro-
        phy
     D. Extra-renal pelvis

107. Pseudo-sludge can be demon-
     strated as a result of:
     A. hematobilia.
     B. side-lobe artifacts.
     C. slice thickness artifact.
     D. B and C

108. Of the following statements
     about pediatric pancreatogra-
     phy, which statement con-
     cerning the pancreas is
     incorrect?
     A. Normally more hypoechoic
        compared to adults
     B. Normally more hyper-
        echoic compared to adults
     C. Trauma is the most signif-
        icant cause of pancreatitis
     D. Pancreatitis is less com-
        mon in children than
        adults

109. The clinical constellation of
     acute right upper quadrant
     (RUQ) pain referred to the

shoulder, nausea and vomiting, and jaundice are classic clinical symptoms of:
A. adenomyomatosis.
B. cholecystitis.
C. pancreatitis.
D. Caroli's disease.

110. Which of the following statements is *untrue* regarding Wilms' tumor?
A. May displace pelvocalyceal system
B. Peak incidence at 13 years of age
C. May invade the IVC, or renal vein
D. Hypertension and anemia present in advanced stage tumors

111. The _____ is an extension of the head of the pancreas that is frequently mistaken for pathology.
A. lingual process
B. uncinate process
C. clinoid process
D. styloid process

112. The main portal vein (MPV) is formed by the splenic vein (SV) and superior mesenteric vein (SMV), behind the neck of the pancreas. The diameter of the MPV should be measured at its origin just superior to the confluence of the SMV and SV, and is considered normal if the diameter is less than:
A. 13 mm.
B. 15 mm.
C. 17 mm.
D. 19 mm.

113. Which of the following is *not* a node-bearing area of the retroperitoneum?
A. Iliac
B. Hypogastric
C. Hypergastric
D. Para-aortic

114. Which of the following statements concerning splenic anatomy and physiology is *untrue?*
A. It is retroperitoneal
B. Its hilus often touches the tail of the pancreas
C. It converts iron from hemoglobin
D. It is a source of lymphocytes

115. Portal lymphadenopathy is associated with all of the following conditions *except:*
A. lymphoma.
B. hemangioma.
C. inflammation.
D. metastases.

116. What causes recanalization of the umbilical vein?
A. Hepatocellular carcinoma
B. Portal hypertension
C. Cirrhosis
D. Pancreatitis

117. Besides obstruction of the cystic duct, which of the following conditions may produce a noncontracting gallbladder, even after administration of a fatty meal or IV cholecystokinin?
A. Diabetes and pancreatitis
B. IV hyperalimentation or prolonged fasting

C. Oral cholinergic drug therapy

D. All of the above

118. Which of the following substances makes it possible to sonographically demonstrate the various fissures and ligaments within the liver parenchyma?

A. Collagen and adipose tissue

B. Muscle

C. Blood

D. Interstitial fluid

119. Serous or transudative ascites can be differentiated from subcapsular liver hematomas by observing:

A. limited movement of the fluid.

B. presence of reverberation echoes.

C. failure to respond to respiration.

D. all of the above

120. What is the major disadvantage associated with scanning the kidneys in only sagittal and transverse planes while the patient lies in the prone position?

A. Sound beam travels tangential to medial and lateral aspect of the kidneys

B. Increased interference from gas and fat

C. Decreased transmission because of rib and muscularity of the back

D. Increased interference from air-filled bowel

121. Which of the following is *not* a benefit accrued when studying the caudate lobe and its vasculature?

A. Significant caudate lobe changes can be seen in patients with cirrhosis and Budd-Chiari syndrome.

B. Can affect surgical planning in subtotal hepatectomies

C. Caudate lobe maintains its own blood supply

D. Atrophy of the caudate lobe with perfusion

122. A 9-year-old female was admitted to the emergency room complaining of extreme pain in the region of McBurney's point, fever, and chills. Stat ultrasound revealed the presence of a complex mass in the right iliac fossa, surrounding an enlarged fluid-filled structure with an edematous double wall. The mass contained reflective echoes with acoustic shadowing. A diagnostic possibility in this child is:

A. pelvic inflammatory disease.

B. inflamed appendix.

C. ruptured appendix.

D. bowel hematoma.

123. What causes the presence of floating gallstones in patients scanned immediately after oral cholecystogram studies?

A. Prolonged fasting

B. Decreased specific gravity of bile

C. Increased specific gravity
   of bile
D. Presence of contrast media

124. An aid to visualizing patho-
logic invasion, displacement,
or compression of the inferior
vena cava is:
A. coronal scanning.
B. erect scanning.
C. Valsalva maneuver.
D. prone patient position.

125. Which of the following statements concerning the pan-
creas is *untrue?*
A. The pancreatic duct lumen is usually largest in
the head of the pancreas
B. Scanning is contraindi-
cated in patients who
have undergone gastro-
scopic examination within
6 hours
C. The superior mesenteric
artery can mimic the pan-
creatic duct
D. A collapsed stomach is
sometimes mistaken for
the pancreatic duct

126. What is the advantage of giving glucagon injections, in
addition to filling the patient's stomach with water, as
a prep for abdominal sonography?
A. Creation of a larger acoustic window
B. Inhibits peristalsis
C. Speeds flow of liquid to
the duodenum
D. Reverses dynamic ileus

127. A 47-year-old female, with a
palpable mid-epigastric mass,
was referred to the ultrasound department for an abdominal survey. She had a
family history of pancreatic
disease. Sonography revealed
a bulging, complex mass containing several large, multi-
loculated, cystic structures.
The mass occupied the junction between the body and
tail of the pancreas. Which of
the following represent the
most likely diagnosis in this
case?
A. Anatomical variant
B. Islet cell tumor
C. Pancreatic cystadenocarcinoma
D. Pancreatic adenocar-
cinoma

CASES AND QUESTIONS

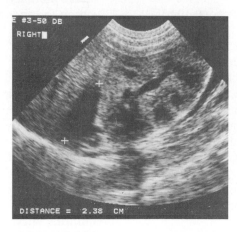

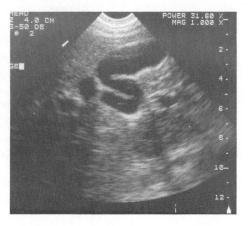

Figure 2-6. Longitudinal scan of the right upper quadrant in a neonate with a history of fetal distress. (Courtesy of Benita Barthel, Ochsner Medical Foundation, New Orleans, Louisiana.)

Figure 2-7. Sagittal scan through the region of the gallbladder. (Courtesy of Linda Novick, Palm Beach Community College, West Palm Beach, Florida.)

A 38-week-old was referred for abdominal ultrasound. The patient was delivered via C-section due to fetal distress (Apgar 7:8), and required back and mask ventilation secondary to persistent bradycardia and poor respiratory efforts. History included known bleeding diathesis and possible intracranial hemorrhage. Laboratory findings were of decreased HGB and HCT; increased PT and PTT. The infant received a transfusion. Reticulocyte count prior to transfusion was 15%, with a maternal Kleihauer-Betke of 0.9%, consistent with ongoing fetal-to-maternal bleed.

128. The area indicated by calipers in Figure 2-6 is consistent with ultrasound findings of:
    A. neuroblastoma.
    B. hydronephrosis.
    C. Wilms' tumor.
    D. adrenal hemorrhage.

A 38-year-old male presented with complaints of right upper quadrant pain, intermittent jaundice, and a small, palpable mass. Lab tests showed slight bilirubin elevation. Sonography revealed a normal-appearing liver without evidence of intrahepatic biliary duct dilatation. The pancreas, kidneys, spleen, and aorta were also noted to be within normal limits. An unusual tortuous, dilated, fluid-filled structure was seen extending from the porta hepatis down to the head of the pancreas. A 1.8 cm cystic area connecting with the common duct was also noted.

129. On the basis of Figure 2-7, the most likely pathology is:
    A. dilated CHD.
    B. dilated CBD.
    C. a choledochocele.
    D. all of the above

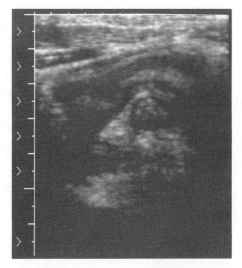

Figure 2-8. Transverse scan of the lower right quadrant. (Courtesy of Kristine Mooney, Rhode Island Hospital, Providence, Rhode Island.)

A 13-year-old female with a history of cystic fibrosis was hospitalized for evaluation of generalized peri-umbilical pain and vomiting. Abdominal ultrasound and barium enema studies were ordered. Scans of the lower right quadrant demonstrated the presence of a persistent structure seen extending from the region of the cecal tip to the proximal ascending colon. A small amount of free fluid was noted in the right paracolic gutter. No other mass was identified, although an incidental finding of gallstones was made.

130. The pathologic process demonstrated in Figure 2-8 is _____, and is most commonly seen in _____.
    A. appendicitis; adolescents
    B. dynamic ileus; adults
    C. intussusception; infants
    D. Crohn's disease; elderly patients

131. Figure 2-8 also demonstrates a classic diagnostic sign, the:
    A. double channel.
    B. doughnut.
    C. target or pseudokidney.
    D. B and C

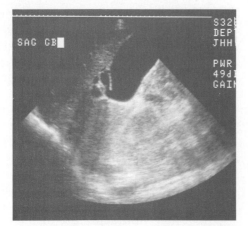

A

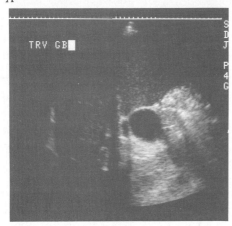

B

Figure 2-9. (*A*) Sagittal and (*B*) transverse scans of the gallbladder. (Courtesy of Noell Blair, Johns Hopkins School of Ultrasound, Baltimore, Maryland.)

Sonograms of the gallbladder and right upper quadrant were ordered for a 31-year-old male AIDS patient who complained of right upper quadrant pain.

132. The gallbladder appeared well dilated and without evidence of stones or sludge. However, in the region of the neck of

the gallbladder, an unusual echo pattern was seen (Fig. 2-9). What is the nature of this finding?
   A. Phrygian cap
   B. Junctional fold
   C. Polyp
   D. Adenomyomatosis

133. What views, in addition to those in Figure 2-9, should be obtained to verify this finding?
   A. Prone
   B. Erect
   C. Decubitus
   D. B and C

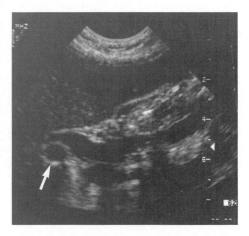

Figure 2-10. Longitudinal image of the right upper quadrant (patient in the left lateral decubitus position). (Courtesy of Alicia Fernandez, Ochsner Medical Foundation, New Orleans, Louisiana.)

An 80-year-old female presented with biliary colic, describing pain radiating to her back after eating fatty foods. She was admitted to the GI service where she underwent an ERCP procedure, followed by abdominal ultrasound.

134. Identify the pathology demonstrated in Figure 2-10.
    A. Cholangitis
    B. Cholelithiasis
    C. Choledocholithiasis
    D. Choledochal cyst

135. Identify the structure indicated by the arrow in Figure 2-10.
    A. Portal vein
    B. Hepatic artery
    C. Hepatic vein
    D. Cystic duct

mm in diameter) demonstrated in Figure 2-11?
    A. Represents a dilated pancreatic duct
    B. Represents a dilated common duct
    C. Is at upper limits of normal size for this structure
    D. B and C

137. What additional pathology is demonstrated in this scan?
    A. Enlarged pancreatic duct
    B. Stone-filled gallbladder
    C. Abnormally echogenic pancreas
    D. Courvoisier gallbladder

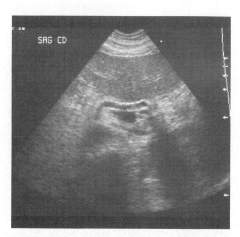

Figure 2-11. Sagittal scan of the right upper quadrant in the region of the gallbladder. (Courtesy of Patricia Revaj, Johns Hopkins Ultrasound School, Baltimore, Maryland.)

This 65-year-old female presented with right upper quadrant pain. Sonographic evaluation of the abdomen was ordered. The liver demonstrated a few tiny liver cysts but no intrahepatic duct dilatation.

136. What is the significance of the echo-free tubular structure (actually measuring 5.3

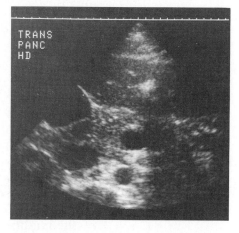

Figure 2-12. Transverse cross-sectional scan through the midline at the level of the pancreatic body. (Courtesy of Stephanie Ellingson, University of Iowa Hospitals and Clinics, Iowa City, Iowa.)

A 21-year-old female is referred to your department with right upper quadrant pain, which is increased during urination.

138. What condition does the sonogram (Fig. 2-12) suggest?
    A. Normal anatomy, includ-

ing inferior vena cava, superior mesenteric vein, abdominal aorta, and super mesenteric artery

B. Duplication of the inferior vena cava

C. Peri-aortic lymphadenopathy

D. Mirror image artifact

139. What is the most likely etiology of this finding?

A. A congenital duplication of the inferior vena cava

B. Myeloproliferative disease

C. Double image artifact caused by beam refraction through the rectus abdominis muscle

D. Misregistration artifact

140. What additional steps should a sonographer take to determine or confirm the etiology of this finding?

A. Image the structures in a sagittal plane

B. Image the structures in an oblique plane

C. Image the structures through a site other than the midline

D. All of the above

141. This finding is most commonly seen with:

A. static scanners.

B. single element real-time transducers.

C. linear-array transducers.

D. annular-array transducers.

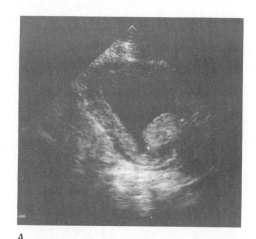

A

B

Figure 2-13. (*A*) Sagittal scan of the bladder. (*B*) Sagittal scan of the right kidney. (Courtesy of Yansheng Wei, SUNY Diagnostic Medical Imaging Program, Brooklyn, New York.)

During a routine physical exam, a 57-year-old male with no significant past medical history was found to have elevated BUN and creatinine laboratory values. The patient admitted to frequent urination at night. The clinical impression was renal insufficiency. Both renal and pelvic sonography were requested to evaluate any underlying pathology.

142. The pathologic process suggested by Figure 2-13 is:
    A. transitional cell carcinoma and hydronephrosis.
    B. BPH and hydronephrosis.
    C. BPH and UTI.
    D. calculus at right ureteropelvic junction.

143. The bladder wall is considered abnormally thickened whenever it measures greater than:
    A. 3 mm.
    B. 3–6 mm.
    C. 4 mm.
    D. 5 mm.

A. Ascites
B. Hepatomegaly
C. Pleural effusion
D. Hydronephrosis

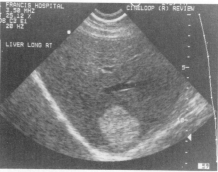

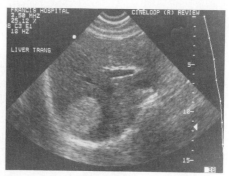

Figure 2-15. (A) Longitudinal and (B) transverse scans of the right upper quadrant demonstrating the presence of a mass within the substance of the liver. (Courtesy of Dayna Landru and Tracy Pfizenmaier, St. Francis School of Diagnostic Medical Sonography, Milwaukee, Wisconsin.)

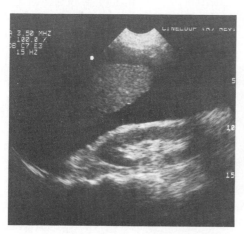

Figure 2-14. Longitudinal scan of the right upper quadrant. (Courtesy of Alicia Fernandez, Ochsner Medical Foundation, New Orleans, Louisiana.)

A 42-year-old white male with a history of cirrhosis presented for abdominal sonography. The patient's chart could not be obtained for further history.

144. What is the pathologic process visible in Figure 2-14?

A 27-year-old female was referred for abdominal sonography to rule out gallstones. No clinical records were available; however, the patient gave a history of long-standing oral contraceptive use.

145. The depicted mass in Figure
     2-15*A,B* most likely repre-
     sents:
     A. hematoma.
     B. bull's-eye lesion.
     C. hemangioma.
     D. echinococcal cyst.

146. Which answer best describes
     the appearance of this mass?
     A. Hypoechoic, with shaggy
        borders
     B. Hypoechoic, with smooth
        borders
     C. Homogeneous, echo-
        dense, with shaggy bor-
        ders
     D. Homogeneous, dense
        mass with sharply defined
        borders

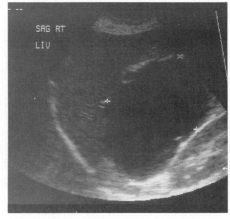

B

Figure 2-16. (*continued*) (*B*) Sagittal
scan of the right upper quadrant.
(Courtesy of Esther London, Johns
Hopkins School of Ultrasound, Baltimore, Maryland.)

The patient is a 65-year-old female
referred for a sonogram of the gallbladder and right upper quadrant to
rule out gallbladder calculi.

147. What pathology is demon-
     strated in the scans in Figure
     2-16?
     A. Subphrenic abscess
     B. Hydronephrosis
     C. Ruptured gallbladder
     D. Hepatic cyst

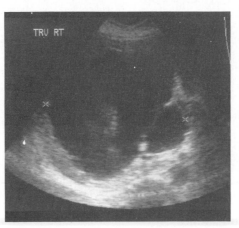

A

Figure 2-16. (*A*) Transverse scan of the
right upper quadrant.

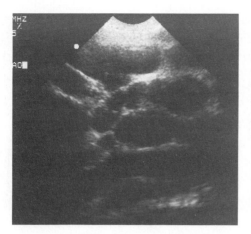

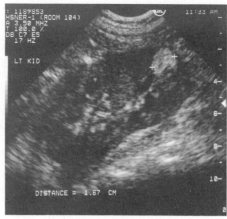

Figure 2-17. Sagittal midline scan selected from an extensive series of abdominal and pelvic sonograms. (Courtesy of Linda Novick, Palm Beach Community College, West Palm Beach, Florida.)

Figure 2-18. Coronal scan of the left kidney. (Courtesy of Benita Barthel, Ochsner Medical Foundation, New Orleans, Louisiana.)

The patient is a 51-year-old male with a known bowel disorder and intractable pain. A 2.8 cm × 3.3 cm × 3.0 cm mass within the liver (between the anterior segment and the right lobe) and marked splenomegaly were demonstrated on the sonographic series. At that time the pancreas and kidneys were described as normal.

The patient is a 61-year-old female with mid-epigastric pain, and fever. Abdominal sonography was performed and demonstrated the presence of a hyperechoic left renal mass. Additional scans throughout the remainder of the abdominal cavity revealed mile splenomegaly, cholelithiasis, and sludge within the gallbladder.

148. Which of the following entities are demonstrated in Figure 2-17?
    A. Mantle sign
    B. Fluid within the stomach
    C. Peri-pancreatic and paravertebral lymphadenopathy
    D. All of the above

149. The calipers in Figure 2-18 are used to indicate the suspected mass area. This structure has the typical sonographic appearance of a (an):
    A. hemangioma.
    B. leukemic infiltrate.
    C. metastases.
    D. angiomyolipoma.

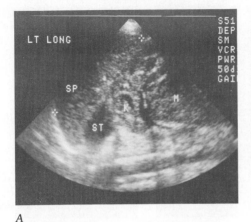

A

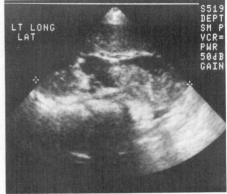

B

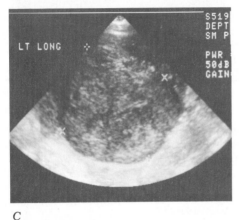

C

Figure 2-19. (*A*) Longitudinal left upper quadrant scan demonstrating a mass and the longitudinal dimension of the spleen (SP, spleen; ST, fluid-filled stomach; M, mass; K, upper pole of left kidney). (*B*) Sagittal scan of the left kidney (calipers indicate left kidney measurement). (*C*) Sagittal section through the medial aspect of the left kidney (calipers indicate measurement of the left kidney mass). (Courtesy of Stephanie Ellingson, University of Iowa Hospitals and Clinics, Iowa City, Iowa.)

The patient is a 15-month-old male who presented with a fever, cold symptoms, and palpable splenomegaly.

150. Figure 2-19*A* demonstrates the following abnormal finding:
    A. splenomegaly.
    B. metastases involving the spleen.
    C. Wilms' tumor.
    D. polycystic kidney disease.

151. The hypoechoic components within the mass demonstrated in Figure 2-19*C* most likely represent:
    A. hemorrhagic and necrotic areas.
    B. multiple cysts consistent with IPKD.
    C. calcifications.
    D. medullary pyramids.

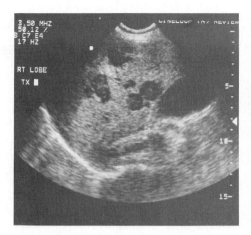

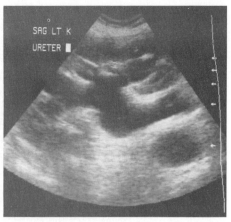

Figure 2-20. Transverse scan of the right upper quadrant. (Courtesy of Jeanie Marchese, Ochsner Medical Foundation, New Orleans, Louisiana.)

Figure 2-21. Sagittal scans of the left kidney and ureter. (Courtesy of Pam Columbo and Carolyn Talley, Johns Hopkins School of Ultrasound, Baltimore, Maryland.)

This 42-year-old white female presented with complaints of nausea, increasing abdominal pain, and dark urine. She has a known history of infiltrating ductal adenocarcinoma of the left breast and metastatic deposits in the brain, lung, and bone. Laboratory findings: increased levels of total bilirubin, direct bilirubin, SGOT, SGPT, LDH, and AP.

152. The liver shown in Figure 2-20 measures 16.52 cm, which is consistent with _____. In addition, the sonographic findings seen in this image are highly suspicious of _____.
    A. hepatic atrophy; hepatitis
    B. abnormally small liver; hepatic cysts
    C. hepatomegaly; hepatic metastatic disease
    D. hyperechoic liver; hemangiomas

Figure 2-21 demonstrates the sonographic appearance of area of the kidney and ureter. Hydronephrosis was noted.

153. What single finding suggests that an obstruction is probably in the distal portion of the urinary tract?
    A. Degree of hydronephrosis
    B. Dilated proximal ureter
    C. Dilated renal pelvis
    D. Presence of cysts

154. Which of the following lab values would be abnormal in a patient with this degree of hydronephrosis?
    A. Decreased creatinine clearance
    B. Elevated creatinine
    C. Increased BUN
    D. All of the above

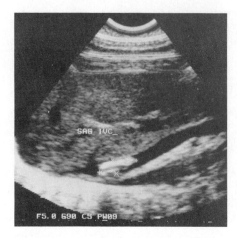

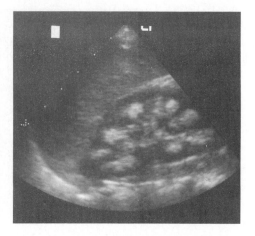

Figure 2-22. Sagittal view of the right upper quadrant. (Courtesy of Sandra Karol, Palm Beach Community College, West Palm Beach, Florida.)

Figure 2-23. Sagittal scan of the right kidney. (Courtesy of Jay Milio and Lance Silwick, Francis Scott Medical Center and Johns Hopkins School of Ultrasound, Baltimore, Maryland.)

Hepatic ultrasound was ordered on a 6-week-old female to rule out hepatomegaly. Examination revealed a normal liver and biliary system. In the upper aspect of the inferior vena cava (Fig. 2-22), a suspicious, discrete, and somewhat echo-dense structure was noted. This finding was duplicated on both longitudinal and transverse scans.

The patient is a 4-year-old male with known chronic heart disease.

156. This renal sonogram (Fig. 2-23) demonstrates a classic sonographic example of:
    A. acute glomerulonephritis.
    B. renal artery stenosis.
    C. nephrocalcinosis.
    D. hydronephrosis.

155. The findings presented here are highly suggestive of:
    A. global enlargement of the IVC.
    B. intraluminal abscess.
    C. intraluminal thrombus.
    D. intraluminal embolus.

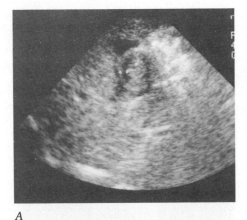

A

B

Figure 2-24. (*A*) Oblique scan through the upper abdomen. (*B*) Repeat scan through the same area utilizing a fluid-filled stomach as an acoustic window. (Courtesy of Stephanie Ellingson, University of Iowa Hospitals and Clinics, Iowa City, Iowa.)

This 2-month-old male was referred for abdominal ultrasound. The infant had a history of multiple episodes of emesis and at least one episode of projectile vomiting.

157. The calipers seen on Figure 2-24*A* demonstrate the measurement of:
    A. the gallbladder.
    B. the pylorus of the stomach.
    C. the right kidney.
    D. a liver mass.

158. The structure demonstrated in Figure 2-24*B* most likely represents _____, and the hyperechoic lines demonstrated within the center of this structure represent _____.
    A. hypertrophic pyloric stenosis; mucosa
    B. duodenal atresia; muscularis mucosa
    C. thick walled gallbladder; gallbladder lumen
    D. renal hypertrophy; calcifications

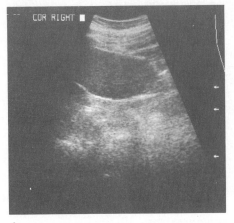
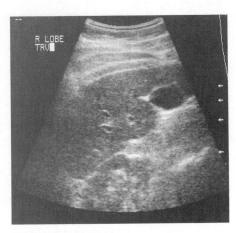

A   B

Figure 2-25. (A) Coronal and (B) transverse scans of the right quadrant. (Courtesy of Yvonne Hoeflich and Gale White, Johns Hopkins School of Ultrasound, Baltimore, Maryland.)

The patient is a 32-year-old, asymptomatic female, whose insurance company ordered a pre-policy physical examination. She is referred for abdominal ultrasound (Fig. 2-25) to rule out hepatomegaly because of the palpation of a right-sided "mass."

159. What is the most likely finding in this patient?
    A. Hepatosplenomegaly
    B. Chronic hepatitis
    C. Reidel's lobe
    D. Hydatid cyst

160. For diagnostic confirmation in this patient, the sonographer should also image the:
    A. porta hepatis.
    B. left lobe of the liver.
    C. Morrison's pouch.
    D. ligamentum teres.

ANSWERS

1. B. Fever and an increase in the number of white blood cells are common manifestations of infection. Most organs respond to infection with the formation of an abscess. In the involved area, the organ becomes swollen and more sonolucent. Local tenderness is also present.[2, 9, 11, 20, 22]

2. D. The presence of structures such as bone, air, and barium are known to inhibit the transmission of sound. For this reason ultrasound should always be performed before any barium or endoscopic studies in the area of interest. To a lesser degree, the loss of tissue fluid associated with dehydration or prolonged radiation therapy may also contribute to the production of a suboptimal examination. Sonographers must be alert to such potential problems and take whatever patient preparations or positional changes that are necessary to obtain the highest-quality diagnostic studies.[2, 11]

3. C. Cavernous hemangiomas are large, fluid-filled arteriovenous malformations composed of large networks of vascular endothelium-lined spaces filled with red blood cells. A capillary hemangioma is a smaller benign overgrowth of capillaries that frequently presents as a highly echogenic focal lesion.[14]

4. B. Late manifestations of cirrhosis include splenomegaly, jaundice, ascites, GI bleeding (varices), portal hypertension, and reopening of the umbilical vein.[19] (Courtesy of Benita Barthel, Ochsner Medical Foundation, New Orleans, Louisiana.)

5. B. Cysts may also be demonstrated in the liver in approximately 33% of patients, the pancreas in 10%, and the spleen in 5%. In rare cases, cystic changes are also present in the ovaries, testes, uterus, thyroid, and lungs.[2, 11]

6. 1. C, 2. H, 3. E, 4. A, 5. F, 6. B, 7. D, 8. G[7, 18]

7. C. Jaundice is a condition characterized by yellowness of the skin, mucous membranes, and secretions due to bile pigments in the blood. Congenital or acquired obstructions of the biliary system are the most common causes. Jaundice is a result, not a cause, of biliary cirrhosis.[19] (Courtesy of Benita Barthel, Ochsner Medical Foundation, New Orleans, Louisiana.)

8. C. The appearance of retroperitoneal fibrosis on ultrasound is usually that of a hypoechoic midline mass. This dense, fibrous tissue

proliferation is a plaque-like or a bulky mass (2–6 cm thick) and is generally confined to the para-vertebral and central regions. It may be associated with bilateral ureteral obstruction as it envelops structures rather than displacing them. Patients may present with back, abdominal, or flank pain. There may be signs of weight loss, hypertension, and accompanying nausea and vomiting.[2]

9. B. The sandwich sign describes the sonographic appearance of enlarged lymph nodes lying anterior and posterior to the superior mesenteric artery and the mesenteric sheath in the mesentery.[20]

10. A. The main lobar fissure, located between the gallbladder neck and the right portal vein, divides the liver into the intrahepatic right and left lobes.[2,4]

11. D. The primary branching of the portal vein and hepatic artery at the porta hepatis establishes two right segments, two left segments, and the caudate lobe of the liver.[4] (Courtesy of Mark Houck, Orange Coast College, Costa Mesa, California.)

12. B. The highest-frequency transducer should be used to produce the optimal resolution. If adequate penetration to the posterior liver cannot be obtained with a high-frequency transducer, a lower-frequency transducer should be used. In most adults the liver is examined using a 3 to 3.5 MHz transducer.[2]

13. B. Fusion of the metanephros across the midline during fetal development results in the common anomaly of horseshoe kidney. There is usually parenchymal or fibrous tissue fusion of the lower poles, which results in an abnormal axis of the "kidney," with the upper poles more lateral than the fused lower poles. The kidney will be low in position, as complete ascent is impeded by the root of the inferior mesenteric artery.[22] Generally asymptomatic and capable of normal function, horseshoe kidneys can be associated with hydronephrosis, infection, or calculus formation. Patients are often referred for evaluation of a pulsatile abdominal mass. Scans are then carried out to confirm or deny the presence of an aortic aneurysm, pancreatic enlargement, or lymphadenopathy.[11]

14. D. Liver function tests in patients with metastatic lesions of the liver are frequently abnormal. Increases in alkaline phosphatase, SGOT, and SGPT are common. An increase in alpha-fetoprotein (a carcino-embryonic antigen) is often noted in cases of liver metastases.[19] (Courtesy of Benita Barthel, Ochsner Medical Foundation, New Orleans, Louisiana.)

15. 1. M, 2. G, 3. O, 4. I, 5. K, 6. A, 7. L, 8. C, 9. B, 10. D, 11. H, 12. N, 13. P, 14. F, 15. J, 16. E[7, 18]

16. D. Vascular compromise following gallbladder inflammation invariably leads to gangrenous changes, as the cystic artery is an end artery. Teefey et al. observed a new sonographic finding—striated (heterogeneous) thickening of the gallbladder wall—as well pericholecystic fluid collections, intraluminal membranes, and mass-like projections to be suspect for gangrenous cholecystitis.[24]

17. D. Malignancies originating within the lymphatic system are called lymphomas, a questionable term because it suggests a benign condition. Lymphomas can be roughly divided into Hodgkin's disease and non-Hodgkin's lymphomas.[5] The etiology of Hodgkin's disease is not known. The disease presents some of the features of a neoplasm but inflammatory changes are also an intrinsic component, so that the possibility of an infective origin still remains. The current, most widely held view is that it is a malignant neoplasm (Hodgkin's mononuclear cells). Inflammatory and immunological changes (Reed-Sternberg cells) are interpreted as being secondary to the neoplastic proliferation.[6]

18. C[2, 4]

19. A. Sonographically, the appearance of adrenal hemorrhage depends on the age of the hemorrhage. Initially, hemorrhage appears echogenic, becoming progressively more sonolucent as it liquifies. Within a short time the affected gland usually shrinks rapidly and develops a calcific rim. As the gland continues to decrease in size the calcifications become more compact, eventually conforming to the triangular configuration of the normal gland.[11, 19] (Courtesy of Benita Barthel, Ochsner Medical Foundation, New Orleans, Louisiana.) Lymphocytes develop within the white pulp of the spleen for use in defense against disease. Another splenic function is the removal or destruction of aged red cells and the metabolism of their iron for reuse in hemoglobin.[1]

20. A. The portal vein margins are highly reflective because of their high collagen content and proximity to hepatic arteries and bile ducts.[11]

21. A. The neck of the gallbladder bears a fixed anatomic relationship to the main lobar fissure and right portal vein.[2]

22. C. Tumors arising in the lymph nodes spread to other nodes, bone marrow, and spleen. Eventually the spread can be generalized and

many organs may be infiltrated (e.g., heart, CNS, kidney, liver, and lungs). Ecotaxis refers to a "homing instinct" that causes spread first to the contralateral organ.[6]

23. D. The crus of the diaphragm may be misread as a normal right adrenal gland. The crus is a tubular structure that lies medial to the adrenal location. On the left side, many structures converge in the vicinity of the adrenal. The esophagastric junction, the tail of the pancreas, splenic vessels, the stomach, and lobulations of the spleen or kidney can all mimic the adrenal. Always identify or rule out a normal structure before deciding that adrenal pathology is present.[20] A large fatty neoplasm in the liver or right adrenal (e.g., liver lipoma, adrenal myelolipoma) will cause apparent disruption of the diaphragmatic echo. This is an artifact caused by changes in the propagation speed of the sound beam through the fatty tumor.[22] In cases of renal agenesis, the adrenal gland relaxes down into the empty renal fossa. Although it may resemble the kidney, failure to demonstrate the normal sonographic pattern of the adrenal gland and the lack of a typical renal collecting system echo pattern should prevent such recognition errors.

24. A. A direct increase in bilirubin is associated with a variety of conditions capable of producing obstruction, such as hepatocellular disease, obstructive liver disease, or gram-negative septicemia. Indirect bilirubin increases in diseases that cause hemolysis, such as hemolytic jaundice.[2, 11]

25. B. The liver is composed of hexagonal or cylindric lobules constructed around a central vein. At each of the six corners of a lobule the portal tract or triad can be found, consisting of a branch of the hepatic artery, a branch of the portal vein, and a bile duct.[11]

26. D. In severe rejection the renal sinus "blends" with the adjacent parenchyma so that the boundary between the two compartments cannot be identified. Most often the renal allograft is placed retroperitoneally in an oblique orientation into the recipient's contralateral iliac fossa, anterior to the psoas muscle and iliac veins. The superficial position of the transplanted kidney allows excellent sonographic delineation of its anatomy and pathology so that the highest-resolution transducers are preferred. Signs of acute rejection include enlargement of the renal pyramids, decreased echogenicity (edema), and congestion and hemorrhage of the interstitial tissue.[9, 11]

27. 1. H, 2. P, 3. F, 4. B, 5. O, 6. C, 7. J, 8. A, 9. M, 10. K, 11. G, 12. L, 13. D, 14. N, 15. I, 16. E[7, 18]

28. D. Laboratory findings associated with acute pancreatitis are leukocytosis due to inflammation, tissue necrosis, and infection. Hyperglycemia, resulting from the loss of insulin normally secreted into the blood stream, is common. Extremely high fasting blood sugars (FBS) are seen in acute pancreatitis, since insulin destined for the blood stream leaks out of the damaged pancreatic cells and is destroyed by enzymes released from other damaged pancreatic cells. Serum amylase elevation occurs with the leakage of amylase from damaged pancreatic cells and its absorption into the blood stream by surrounding blood vessels. Serum bilirubin and liver enzymes are often elevated, primarily because of bile duct obstruction caused by pressure from the swollen pancreas. AFP (alpha fetoprotein) is associated with the development of liver neoplasms and is unrelated to pancreatic function.[5]

29. C. Ascitic fluid will collect in the most dependent portion of the body. One of the most obvious ascites collection sites is the subhepatic space (Morrison's pouch).[4, 11]

30. C. The quadrate lobe lies between the fissure for the ligamentum teres and the gallbladder fossa, anterior to the porta hepatis.[2] According to Sanders, the term quadrate lobe is now considered obsolete.[20]

31. C. An erroneous diagnosis of hydronephrosis may be made in patients with bladder over-distention. Postvoid scans of the bladder and kidneys should be made whenever hydronephrosis appears present.[20]

32. B. As lymph nodes enlarge they may take on an irregular appearance, and may drape (mantle) over the prevertebral vessels (para-aortic nodes). Such nodes have lobular, smooth, or scalloped appearances; if mesenteric adenopathy is also present, they characteristically "sandwich" (form on either side of) the mesenteric sheath in two large groups.[9]

33. D. In the fasting state, the upper limits of normal is 3 mm. In the postprandial state, the gallbladder wall will appear thicker but should still measure 3 mm or less in thickness.[22]

34. B. Prothrombin time (PT) is a test used to determine pathologic deficiency of clotting factors due either to liver dysfunction or absence of vitamin K. When correlated with parenchymal disease, scarred, nonfunctioning liver tissue does not produce prothrombin.[11]

35. C. Bladder diverticulae are pouchlike extensions of the bladder produced by herniation through a weak bladder muscle wall. Trauma and bleeding are not associated with this condition.[2,11,20]

36. D. The liver receives nutrients via the hepatic artery and portal vein. The portal vein supplies 50% to 60% of the oxygen required by hepatocytes.[2]

37. D. Autosomal dominant, or adult polycystic kidney disease, is a disorder in which the symptomatic features of the disease are expressed in one or both of the parents of an affected person. Autosomal recessive, or infantile polycystic kidney disease, is a disorder that requires that both parents of an affected individual possess the gene causing the disease.[13]

38. D. Accessory spleens are common and usually found incidentally. They are usually located at the hilum of the spleen. Lymphoma is a common involvement of the spleen but is difficult to detect on sonograms. Cavernous hemangioma is a rare splenic finding that produces an inhomogeneous echogenic pattern.[2]

39. B. The sonographic spectrum of abscesses is very wide. Some appear echo-free or hypoechoic and may resemble liquifying hematomas or cysts, some have septations, filaments, or internal debris, simulating hydatid disease, and occasionally, bubbles of gas appear as highly reflective echoes.[22]

40. C. Neuroblastoma is the most common adrenal tumor of childhood and, after Wilms' tumor, the second most common cause of intra-abdominal tumor in children. Seventy-five percent occur in children under 4 years with occurrence uncommon after age 8. Symptoms include hyperirritability and failure to thrive. Unlike Wilms' tumor, neuroblastoma spreads rapidly beyond the confines of the adrenal gland, often crossing the midline in the abdomen. Calcification is a common finding in neuroblastoma.[2,9,11,22]

41. B. The prostate gland is an oval-shaped retroperitoneal structure comprised of five lobes: the anterior, middle, posterior, and two lateral lobes.[2,9]

42. C. The role of ultrasonography in hepatitis is to evaluate parenchymal changes. In the acute phase of hepatitis the appearance ranges from normal to hypoechoic. On the other hand, fibrosis resulting from chronic hepatitis produces a hyperechoic texture.[11]

43. D. In most cases of cystic fibrosis the pancreas will appear hyper-echoic, probably due to increased fibrotic and fatty infiltration. Chronic pancreatitis is characterized by increased echogenicity due to fibrotic changes, fatty changes, and the development of calcifications.[2]

44. B. Normal ducts are thin-walled. Only the internal dimensions of ducts should be measured.[2,11]

45. 1. K, 2. F, 3. L, 4. C, 5. A, 6. E, 7. D, 8. H, 9. B, 10. I, 11. J, 12. G[7,18]

46. C. Sound traveling through fluid alone encounters no density change sufficient to cause reflection and the production of echoes. (Courtesy of Benita Barthel, Ochsner Medical Foundation, New Orleans, Louisiana.)

47. A. The sonographic echo pattern of fatty infiltrative disease, cirrhosis, or hepatitis depends on the severity of the condition. One sonographic finding is that of focal sparing of the caudate lobe, which may occur in an otherwise diffuse process, making the normal tissue appear as a hypoechoic defect.[11]

48. D. In the setting of acute trauma, the sonographer must examine the pelvis, Morrison's pouch, and the flanks for the presence of free blood. Hemoperitoneum may be suggested by the sonographic demonstration of fluid in the lesser and greater sac on both sides of the gastrosplenic ligament. Weill describes this finding as the butterfly sign.[2,11]

49. C. The upper limits of normal size are 4 to 5 mm for the CHD and 6 to 8 mm for the CBD.[2]

50. B. The target or bull's-eye pattern—a discrete round or oval abnormality with dense central echoes and an anechoic periphery—is a characteristic sonographic feature of stomach and bowel abnormalities. The target pattern has been described in cases of malignant tumors but also in Crohn's disease, intramural hematoma, pancreatitis, and radiation enteritis.[3,11]

51. D. Stones may appear to float. If a patient has had a recent cholecystogram, the contrast raises the specific gravity of the bile and can cause this phenomenon.[2]

52. D. The caliber of the hepatic veins becomes greater as they course toward the diaphragm and the IVC.[11]

53. C. Kaposi's sarcoma is the most common hepatic tumor in AIDS patients at autopsy. However, it is difficult to diagnose by percutaneous liver biopsy. Most likely this is because of its subcapsular and periportal distribution. Since such areas would likely escape sampling by routine blind biopsy, diagnostic ultrasound plays an important role in the evaluation of these patients.[26]

54. A. The features of Mirizzi syndrome include the presence of an impacted stone in the cystic duct or gallbladder neck, partial mechanical obstruction of the common hepatic duct by compression or inflammatory reaction, and dilatation of the common hepatic duct about the level of the gallstone with normal duct below the stone.[2,11,22]

55. C. The cortex and renal pyramids together constitute the renal parenchyma, which contains the basic histologic and functional unit of the kidney, the nephron.[2,4,11]

56. C. Hepatic cysts may be congenital, traumatic, parasitic, or inflammatory in origin. Congenital cysts may arise from development defects in the formation of bile ducts. They may vary in size from 3 cm to 13 liters. They usually do not cause liver enlargement and are rarely palpable. Hepatic cysts are usually asymptomatic but occasionally cause epigastric pain. The right lobe is affected twice as often as the left.[2,11]

57. C. The sonographic features of chronic cholecystitis are a small contracted gallbladder with stones and a thick, fibrous, echogenic wall. With careful technique, a wall-echo (stone) -shadow triad or "double-arc" shadow sign can be observed. The first arc or curved echogenic line represents the thickened gallbladder wall; the second arc is from the surface of the stone followed by posterior acoustic shadowing.[2,11,22]

58. D. Sonography can detect both benign and malignant focal abnormalities. The presence of calcification suggests that the primary tumor is a mucinous adenocarcinoma, such as those derived from colon or ovary.[14]

59. D. If splenomegaly is present the liver should be examined for evidence of diffuse liver disease and any portal and splenic vein enlargement indicating portal hypertension. Sonographers should also

note whether any nodes are present in association with the splenomegaly that might indicate the presence of lymphoma.[2,20]

60. B. Normally, the echogenicity of the pancreas is equal to or greater
    than that of the liver, but this depends on the patient's age and
    body habitus.[2,4,11,22]

61. C. Simple, uncomplicated renal cysts are the most common mass
    in the adult kidney. They are benign, fluid-filled, nonneoplastic cys-
    tic masses of unknown etiology. They are usually asymptomatic and
    require no treatment. Simple uncomplicated cortical cysts are un-
    common in infants and children.[22] The prevalence of such cysts is
    uncommon before age 40, increasing markedly thereafter to reach
    approximately 50% for persons older than 55 years.[11] Simple renal
    cysts consist of smooth walls, no internal echoes, and acoustic en-
    hancement posterior. They usually are cortical and bulge through
    the renal capsule. They may cause partial obstruction of the collect-
    ing system.[2]

62. D. Cirrhosis is a diffuse process characterized by fibrosis and con-
    version of normal liver architecture into structurally abnormal nod-
    ules. The essential feature in generalized advance cirrhosis is of
    diffuse fibrosis and irreversible scarring.[2]

63. B. The main pancreatic duct (duct of Wirsung) is considered di-
    lated when its internal diameter exceeds 2 mm (within the pancre-
    atic body).[2,11]

64. D. Increased cortical echogenicity can be caused by a large number
    of renal pathologies including acute and chronic glomerulonephri-
    tis, diffuse infiltrating lymphoma, and infantile polycystic kidney
    disease.[22]

65. B. Sludge produces a homogeneous, low-amplitude echo pattern
    that tends to layer dependently. True sludge often forms a straight
    horizontal line that moves slowly with changes in patient position.
    Sludge will not produce acoustic shadowing.[11] The presence of
    sludge implies the formation of a precipitate and should not be
    regarded as normal. Sludge is sometimes a precursor to gallstone
    disease.[22]

66. A. The renal cortex is homogeneous and slightly less echogenic
    than the liver. The renal pyramids are anechoic in appearance. The
    renal sinus and peri-renal fat appear very echogenic.[2]

67. B. Biliary sludge, in ultrasound parlance, has come to mean echogenic bile caused by calcium bilirubinate or cholesterol crystals.[22]

68. C. Calcification of all or part of the gallbladder wall is called *porcelain gallbladder.* It is a relatively rare manifestation of chronic cholecystitis and is frequently asymptomatic. It is associated with a high incidence of gallbladder carcinoma.[11] Hyperechoic mural foci may arise from (1) calcification within the walls of the gallbladder (porcelain gallbladder), (2) small intramural calculi (within the Rokitansky-Aschoff sinuses), (3) calculi adherent to the mucosa, (4) calcified cholesterol polyps, or (5) gas within the gallbladder wall (emphysematous cholecystitis).[22]

69. B. According to Shimamoto et al., color Doppler imaging provides useful information for characterizing intratumoral blood flow. The Doppler signals and resistive index of tumor vessels becomes lower as vessels progress into the center of a lesion.[23]

70. C. The left renal vein arises medially from the renal hilus and flows from the left kidney posterior to the SMA and anterior to the abdominal aorta and inferior vena cava. It is longer than the right renal vein and accepts branches from the left adrenal, left gonadal, and lumbar veins.[2, 4, 18] (Courtesy of Cheryl Powell, Orange Coast College, Costa Mesa, California.)

71. C. It is useful to determine the caudate lobe width and divide it by the width of the right lobe, as seen on a transverse section. Cirrhosis is diagnosed if the ratio is greater than 0.65; if the ratio is less than 0.60, cirrhosis is unlikely.[2, 11]

72. A. According to Sauerbrei et al., adenomyomatosis is thought to be a noninflammatory intrinsic disease of the gallbladder wall, characterized by hyperplasia and thickening of the mucosa and muscular layer and by intramural diverticula. Consequently, there would be no obstruction to biliary flow.[22]

73. C. The blood supply to the pancreas is provided by branches of the gastroduodenal, splenic, and superior mesenteric arteries, all of which should be identified during the examination process.[4, 11] (Courtesy of Amy Stillman, Orange Coast College, Costa Mesa, California.)

74. B. Late manifestations of cirrhosis include splenomegaly, jaundice, ascites, GI bleeding (varices), portal hypertension, and reopening of the umbilical vein.[19] (Courtesy of Benita Barthel, Ochsner Medical Foundation, New Orleans, Louisiana.)

75. C. Obstruction to the hepatic venous outflow tract by thrombus or tumor can produce the associated clinical features of abdominal pain, jaundice, hematemesis, ascites, hepatomegaly, and liver function abnormalities indicative of hepatocellular dysfunction. Collectively, these findings are known as the Budd-Chiari syndrome.[11]

76. C. Gallbladder metastases are not as rare as was once thought. The most common tumor to metastasize to the gallbladder is malignant melanoma, usually by embolic hematogenous spread. The clinical presentation can mimic acute or chronic gallbladder inflammation.[11] With gallbladder metastases, calculi are usually absent.[22]

77. D. Up to 80% of patients on chronic hemodialysis will develop multiple small cysts within the native kidneys. Between 8% and 20% of these patients develop renal neoplasms. The natural history is not well understood. Cysts and tumor usually occur after several years of dialysis.[4, 22] (Courtesy of Angela Tyvog, Orange Coast College, Costa Mesa, California.)

78. A. Hydrops occurs with distention of the gallbladder, invariably due to total obstruction of the cystic duct. The trapped bile is resorbed and the gallbladder is filled with clear mucinous secretion derived from the gallbladder wall. The hydropic gallbladder is tense and enlarged and the wall is thin.[2]

79. C. Para-pelvic cysts are parenchymal cysts that bulge into the central sinus of the kidney. They may cause extrinsic compression of the collecting system or mass effect on excretory urography. Peripelvic cysts are lymphatic cysts in the central sinus. They have an identical appearance to and cannot be distinguished from para-pelvic cysts.[22]

80. C. Moderate splenomegaly is seen in collagen diseases or autoimmune disorders. However, massive splenomegaly can be seen in patients with chronic malaria, hematologic disorders such as chronic granulocytic leukemia, and malignant lymphoma.[22] A small, nonfunctional spleen is associated with repeated infarction as occurs with sickle-cell anemia.[11]

81. C. Downward displacement of the SMA is most often associated with the development of a pancreatic neoplasm.[2]

82. B. Diffuse wall thickening may be stimulated by a contracted gallbladder. True wall thickening is most commonly caused by non-inflammatory edema (extrinsic causes) and inflammation (intrinsic

gallbladder disease). Uncommon causes include tumor infiltration, varices secondary to portal hypertension, and adenomyomatosis (often focal or segmental).[4,22] Gallbladder wall thickness may help distinguish between malignant and cirrhotic ascites. If the wall is nonthickened and single-layered, the ascites are usually malignant. If the wall is thickened and double-layered, the ascites are usually cirrhotic.[10] With hydrops of the gallbladder the gallbladder is tense and enlarged and the wall is thin.[2]

83. D. Blood flow in the splenic vessels, at the splenic hilus and adjacent to the pancreatic body, is easily demonstrated by pulsed-wave Doppler and color Doppler ultrasound. The flow in the splenic vein is similar to the portal vein flow, demonstrating continuous flow and low velocity. The flow in the splenic artery demonstrates a systolic peak and low-velocity flow toward the spleen in diastole.[22]

84. C. The extension of renal malignancies into the inferior vena cava occurs through the renal vein in 5% to 6% of cases. Duplex Doppler or color Doppler is valuable in showing the mass, narrowing, or complete occlusion of the renal vein or inferior vena cava. However, with renal vein and IVC involvement, angiography prior to surgery affords a more complete picture of the extent of involvement.[11,22]

85. B. According to Lewis, sonography can detect both benign and malignant focal abnormalities. Many malignant tumors may simulate benign tumors or inflammatory masses. Since hepatocellular carcinoma may have a varied sonographic appearance similar to metastases, it may be difficult to distinguish the primary tumor from hepatic metastases. In this case, the presence of portal vein invasion (most common in hepatomas) makes hepatocellular carcinoma the most likely diagnosis; however, confirmation with CT, angiography, or histologic examination is required.[14]

86. D. When there is a sharp kink near the distal end of the gallbladder, a partial thick septum is evident in the ultrasound scan. This is called a *Phrygian cap*, and it is not clinically significant. More commonly one sees a fold in the neck of the gallbladder, which is also clinically insignificant.[22]

87. 1. D, 2. H, 3. A, 4. G, 5. K, 6. I, 7. B, 8. J, 9. C, 10. E, 11. L, 12. F[7,18]

88. D. AST, or aspartate aminotransferase, is an enzyme that appears in all tissues, but in largest amounts in cells that use the most energy, such as liver, heart, and skeletal muscles. AST is released with

injury to the cells and is most commonly associated with liver diseases (i.e., hepatitis, cirrhosis) or trauma.[11]

89. C. In general, pancreatic neoplasms represent a localized change in pancreatic echogenicity. The echo pattern appears hypoechoic or less echogenic than the normal liver and pancreas.[2]

90. C. Viral hepatitis may be caused by type A, type B, or non-A non-B virus. In acute hepatitis, ultrasound demonstrates hypoechoic liver parenchyma, mild liver enlargement, and hyperechoic portal vein walls (compared with normal). The hypoechoic parenchyma may be caused by swelling of hepatocytes and hyperechoic portal vein walls by inflammatory and fibrous changes in and around the walls of the portal vein radicles.[22]

91. D. Surgical clips adjacent to the bile duct from previous cholecystectomy may be mistaken for intraductal calculi or gas. Similarly, gas within the bowel lying beside the bile duct (especially when the duct is tortuous) can give the appearance of a calculus in the common duct.[22] Junctional folds or the valves of Heister can mimic an echogenic focus with distal shadowing.[11]

92. A. Most people, after a cholecystectomy, have a normal caliber bile duct (i.e., 6 mm or less in internal anteroposterior diameter). In a few patients the duct dilates beyond its presurgical size.[22]

93. C. The intraperitoneal subphrenic spaces are created by folding of the peritoneum in the hepatic region. Both the right and left anterior subphrenic spaces lie between the diaphragm and the liver, one on each side of the falciform ligament.[2, 11, 22]

94. B. Air in the biliary tree (pneumobilia) can result from surgical procedures, such as anastomosis of the biliary tree to the bowel (Roux-en-Y procedures), papillectomy, etc.; or nonsurgical causes, such as gallstone ileus or patulous sphincter of Oddi in an elderly person allowing air from bowel to reflux into the biliary tree. ERCP (endoscopic retrograde cholangiopancreatography) which involves the injection of contrast into the common bile duct (and pancreatic duct) through a catheter that has been inserted into the papilla of Vater via an endoscope positioned in the duodenum, is unlikely to produce air within the biliary system.[11]

95. D. An enlarged and distended Courvoisier gallbladder occurs when there is obstruction distal to the cystic duct due to malignancy (e.g., pancreatic head carcinoma, peri-portal adenopathy). Pancre-

atic adenocarcinoma is the most common type of pancreatic cancer, accounting for 75% of all pancreatic carcinoma of ductal cell origin. Common findings include jaundice, palpable mass in the head/body of the pancreas, and steatorrhea epigastric pain, frequently radiating to the back.[2, 11]

96. D. Echinococcus is a disease caused by the cyst stage of infection by the tapeworm echinococcus, the adult form of which lives in the intestinal tracts of canines. Daughter cysts are separate endocyst formations within the large cyst. Calcified cysts may contain internal and wall calcifications and may appear sonographically hyperechoic with a shadowing focus. Needle aspiration of an echinococcal cyst may cause an anaphylactic reaction. Surgical removal is the treatment of choice.[2, 11, 22]

97. C. Various studies have demonstrated that the internal diameter of the proximal common duct is 4 mm or less in 95% of the population. Diameters greater than 6 mm are considered dilated. The mean diameter increases from 4 to 5 mm for age 30 to 50 years, and from 7 to 8 mm for patients older than 60 years.[22]

98. A. It is believed that blockage of the pancreatic ductules leads to a release of digestive enzymes, which lyse cell walls. As the cell walls are destroyed by proteolytic digestive enzymes, more enzymes are released into the interstitial spaces, precipitating further destruction. Pancreatic pseudocysts are encapsulated collections of the by-products of tissue destruction.[2]

99. D. True enlargement of the liver results from one or more of three main categories of disorder: increase of fluid, increase of cells (fibroblastic, inflammatory, neoplastic) and increased deposition of intracellular or intercellular substance.[16] Right heart failure implies increased pressure and volume of blood in the hepatic venous system and thus increased fluid content in the liver. Ultrasound will demonstrate enlargement of the hepatic veins and inferior vena cava, some generalized liver enlargement (depending on the severity of cardiac compromise), and decreased echogenicity of the liver.[22] The anterior lower edge of the liver is usually an acute, sharp angle. Blunting of the angle suggests the presence of parenchymal disease and is usually associated with enlargement and possible echo pattern abnormalities. This is an important sign, as it may be the only clue to a diffuse liver disorder, other ultrasonic abnormalities being absent.[16]

100. B. Neoplasms of exocrine origin comprise the largest group of pancreatic tumors and include the single most common malignant le-

sion, acinar cell adenocarcinoma. Slightly more than 70% of these lesions occur in the head of the pancreas. The remainder occur equally in the body or tail. Mucinous cystic adenomas—also referred to as cystadenocarcinomas—are usually large, unilocular, encapsulated masses (although some are rare multilocular lesions), found about 60% of the time in the tail of the pancreas.[11, 16, 22]

101. C. Angiomyolipomas result from the proliferation of smooth muscle and blood vessels along with microaneurysms and various amounts of adipose tissue. These benign masses, which produce hematuria, often occur with tuberous sclerosis. Usually affecting females, angiomyolipomas may occur at any age, but the mean age is 40.[9]

102. B. Duplex pulsed Doppler sonography may be a useful and feasible modality in the follow-up of response to TAE in patients with HCC. The presence of detectable Doppler signals within a lesion after TAE indicates patent tumor vessels. On the other hand, disappearance of detectable Doppler signals after TAE indicates devascularization of the lesion. However, this does not necessarily mean that the patient is completely free of hepatocellular carcinoma.[15]

103. D. Whenever possible, an overnight fast is preferred for at least 6 to 8 hours. The purpose of the fast is threefold: (1) because of the intimate relationship of the biliary system and the pancreas, both are scanned simultaneously; (2) fasting ensures an empty stomach; and (3) fasting reduces bowel gas and allows better visualization of the pancreas. When bowel gas obscures pancreatic visualization, one of the following techniques may be useful: ingestion of water to utilize the stomach as a window, glucagon administered to inhibit peristalsis, administering a fatty meal prior to oral water to decrease peristalsis, and use of methylcellulose prior to fluids allowing increased through transmission.[2]

104. C. The highest-frequency transducer capable of obtaining the best resolution should be selected. For optimal imaging, a multifocus transducer is ideal because of its ability to focus at a range of several depths. However, if such a transducer is unavailable, the demonstration of deep pathology requires sacrificing resolution in order to obtain the deeper penetration provided by lower frequencies.[11]

105. D. Care must be taken not to confuse a pancreatic duct with the splenic vein when the duct is dilated. One way to avoid this mistake is to obtain a transverse scan in which both structures are visualized simultaneously; another is to use color Doppler ultrasound. Occasionally, the posterior wall of the collapsed stomach may be

mistaken for the pancreatic duct. In case of doubt, scanning through a fluid-filled stomach will eliminate this confusion.[22] Other structures that may mimic the pancreatic duct include the splenic artery and retroperitoneal fat.[3]

106. D. Hydronephrosis is a condition in which the renal pelvis becomes dilated due to the obstructed outflow of urine, which may produce renal atrophy. The intrinsic causes of hydronephrosis include calculous, blood clot, tumor, stricture, ureterocele, pyelonephritis, and benign prostatic hypertrophy (BPH). False-positive findings of hydronephrosis include a full or over-distended bladder, postsurgical dilatation, and the presence of an extra-renal pelvis.[2]

107. D. Entities that can mimic sludge are hematobilia or bleeding into the biliary tree.[11] Low-level echoes in the gallbladder may be caused by two types of artifacts: slice thickness and side lobe. To distinguish between real sludge and pseudo-sludge, the patient's position should be changed. Real sludge will move, whereas pseudo-sludge will not move.[22]

108. B. Children have less fat than adults, so the hypoechoic character noted in pediatric patients is a normal finding. Pancreatitis is significantly less common in children than in adults but is not all that rare. The most common cause of pediatric pancreatitis is blunt abdominal trauma.[11]

109. B. The clinical symptoms of cholecystitis are variable and include acute RUQ pain referred to the shoulder (inflammatory exudate tracks up beneath the diaphragm causing irritation of the phrenic nerve); fever, nausea, vomiting; leukocytosis, rigid abdominal pain, and jaundice (25%).[2]

110. B. Wilms' tumor, or nephroblastoma, is a malignant neoplasm arising from within the renal parenchyma. It is one of the most common malignant tumors of childhood, with a peak incidence at 3 years of age. Clinically, the patients experience general malaise, weakness, and failure to thrive. In advanced tumor stages patients suffer from hypertension and anemia. Ultrasound findings are that of a complex echogenic mass capable of displacing the pelvocalyceal system. Nephroblastomas may metastasize to the IVC, renal vein, liver, or peritoneal cavity.[2,9]

111. B. Extending posterior and medial from the head of the pancreas is a beak-like projection of pancreatic tissue, the uncinate process.

The uncinate process may be seen just behind the portal confluence in transverse sections.[11]

112. A. In healthy persons the portal vein diameter is usually less than
     13 mm. It has been proposed that the presence of a larger portal
     vein is suggestive of portal venous hypertension; however, this is
     not a consistent finding.[11]

113. C. There are numerous groups of lymph nodes in the abdominal
     cavity: (1) in the gastric region, along the lesser curvature of the
     stomach; (2) in the mesentery, between layers of mesentery which
     drain the intestines; and (3) alongside the aorta, common iliacs
     and external and internal iliacs, which drain the lower extremities
     and pelvic viscera; also the inguinal and hypogastric regions.[18]
     (Courtesy of Carmen Hunn, Orange Coast College, Costa Mesa,
     California.)

114. A. The spleen is an intraperitoneal structure lying between the left
     hemidiaphragm and stomach. The superior surface is bordered by
     the left hemidiaphragm and the medial surface is bordered by the
     stomach, tail of the pancreas, left kidney, and the splenic flexure of
     the colon.[2]

115. B. Enlarged lymph nodes in the porta hepatis may be due to neo-
     plastic or inflammatory diseases. In ultrasound practice most cases
     are due to metastatic deposits or lymphoma.[22]

116. B. The umbilical vein may reopen to decompress portal hyperten-
     sion by reestablishing communication with the systemic veins
     around the umbilicus. Ten to twenty percent of patients with portal
     hypertension may also have a patent umbilical vein. This structure
     is seen in the falciform ligament as a tubular area of approximately
     3 mm or greater.[2, 11, 22]

117. D. Gallbladder size is generally evaluated after 4 or more hours of
     fasting. Persistent gallbladder enlargement may be caused by pro-
     longed fasting, intravenous hyperalimentation therapy, masses or
     enlargement of the head of the pancreas, diabetes with longstand-
     ing insulin dependency, vagotomy, or obstruction to the cystic or
     common bile ducts.[4, 11, 22]

118. A. The collagen-laden walls of the portal and hepatic veins provide
     veritable specular reflecting road maps of the liver anatomy. The
     echogenic changes between liver parenchyma and organ fat are also
     indicators of the various fissures and ligaments associated with he-
     patic anatomy.[11, 22]

119. C. Subcapsular hematomas show limited change in the shape or location of the "fluid" even after changing the patient to a gravity dependent position. Ascites will flow freely to the most dependent part of the body whenever patient position is changed. Hematomas will respond to changes in patient respiration (e.g., Valsalva maneuver) while ascites will not. Reverberation echoes can appear in *any* large fluid collection.[4, 11, 22]

120. A. All of the factors mentioned present problems, but the most significant problem is the misalignment of the transducer to the lie of the kidneys.[2, 4, 11]

121. D. Knowledge and demonstration of caudate anatomy and localization of its vessels is beneficial because the caudate lobe will show significant changes with cirrhosis and Budd-Chiari syndromes. With cirrhosis, the caudate lobe atrophies; perfusion will cause it to enlarge.[6, 22]

122. C. Perforation of an inflamed appendix is a common complication, occurring most often in children and patients older than 50 years of age. Most often the perforation results in a localized walled-off abscess, but occasionally free intraperitoneal spill may occur, causing severe acute peritonitis. The ultrasound patterns of appendiceal abscess usually appear as a complex mass in the right iliac fossa surrounding a swollen appendix. The mass may contain highly reflective echoes with or without acoustic shadowing, which may represent a fecalith or gas bubbles. Free fluid around the cecum and loss of the echogenic mucosal layer in the fluid-filled appendix may also be seen.[11, 22]

123. C. The contrast agent used during oral cholecystogram studies raises the specific gravity of the bile present within the gallbladder and causes the stones to float to the "surface." Ultrasound studies of the gallbladder should always precede any X-ray contrast study to establish a baseline position of the stones.[4] The presence of both thickened bile and thin, watery bile can also cause the appearance of floating gallstones.[22]

124. C. The demonstration of pathology involving the IVC can be assisted by asking the patient to perform a Valsalva maneuver while the sonographer looks for vessel dilatation below an area of obstruction.[2, 4, 20]

125. C. The superior mesenteric artery runs perpendicular to the pancreas, whereas the pancreatic duct runs parallel within the gland.[4, 7, 20]

126. B. Giving water alone will dilate the stomach; however, glucagon administration will inhibit gastric peristalsis, increasing the time period for using the fluid-filled stomach as an acoustic window.[2, 8, 20]

127. C. Cystadenocarcinomas are relatively rare pancreatic tumors. However, they are more commonly seen in middle-aged women. They may appear similar to a pseudocyst since they typically contain anechoic cysts with good through transmission and easily identifiable internal septations. Whereas males develop pancreatic cancers more commonly in the head of the pancreas, cystadenomas in female patients tend to be found in the region of the tail.[2, 6, 9, 11]

128. D. Abdominal ultrasound revealed a mass density in the region of the right adrenal gland, strongly suggesting adrenal hemorrhage. Follow-up scans were advised to monitor any possible change in the character of the mass. Adrenal hemorrhage in the neonate may be associated with neonatal sepsis or hypoxia, birth trauma affecting the adrenal glands, and bleeding disorders. An aid in differentiating adrenal hemorrhage from neonatal neuroblastoma is the performance of serial ultrasound scans.[19]

129. D. Surgery approximately 1 month following sonography yielded the diagnosis of choledochal cyst. Choledochal cysts are a form of cystic dilatation of the biliary system and usually present as an abdominal mass accompanied by pain, fever, or jaundice. Incidence is greatest in children but the masses may also occur in adults and may be associated with gallstones, pancreatitis, or even cirrhosis. However, the majority of cases are thought to be congenital due to bile reflux. According to Mittelstaedt, choledochal cysts can be described as *Type I*, localized cystic dilatation of the CBD with normal CHD, cystic duct, and gallbladder; *Type II*, as a diverticulum arising from the CBD; *Type III*, an invagination of the CBD (choledochocele) into the duodenum, analogous to a ureterocele in the bladder; and *Type IV*, dilatation of the whole CBD and CHD.[17, 24]

130. C. Intussusception occurs when the proximal loop of the bowel telescopes into the lumen of the adjacent distal portion. Early diagnosis and intervention is critical to prevent bowel obstruction, perforation, peritonitis, or vascular compromise leading to gangrene.[11, 19, 25]

131. D. The appearance of concentric rings (intussuscipiens) in the form of discrete round or oval structures containing dense central echoes (mucosal interfaces) and an anechoic periphery (edematous bowel wall) is the characteristic sonographic feature of stomach and bowel abnormalities. It is variably described as a target, bull's-eye,

doughnut, or pseudokidney sign. Intussusception typically occurs in infants and young children (3 mos.–3 yrs.). However, it is also associated with children older than 3 years who have cystic fibrosis, appendicitis, or who have undergone recent surgery.[2, 11, 19, 25]

132. B. Common anatomical variations of the gallbladder may cause it to fold over on itself or to contain a septum. Septa are usually seen in the region where the neck and body of the gallbladder meet (the junctional fold). If only a portion of the septum is seen on a single scan, it can resemble a gallstone or polyp in the dependent portion of the gallbladder.[20]

133. D. A decubitus or erect view can straighten out a folded gallbladder and correctly identify the suspected stone to be nothing more than a kink.[20]

134. C. The ultrasound study demonstrates a dilated common bile duct (approximately 1 cm) along with common bile duct stones and gallstones. The ERCP revealed two 5-mm common bile duct stones, which were removed. The duct was about 12 mm in size. The patient subsequently underwent laparoscopic cholecystectomy.

135. A. The arrow indicates the specular walls and dilated lumen of the portal vein.

136. D. The 5.3-mm tubular structure represents the common duct which contains no evidence of intraductal stone and is within normal limits for a patient of this age.

137. B. The gallbladder appears to contain numerous small stones and evidence of shadows. Additional scans of the patient's right upper quadrant demonstrated a small right pleural effusion. The pancreas and kidneys were unremarkable in appearance.

138. D. A mirror image artifact of the abdominal aorta and superior mesenteric artery is seen. Such artifacts are often seen when the sound beam encounters a curved structure and duplicates the reflected echo at a deeper level.[12, 19]

139. C. The strong specular reflecting quality of the rectus abdominis muscle is angle-dependent and prone to act like a mirror, creating a double image. This type of artifact will disappear if the scanning angle is changed.[24]

140. D. When dealing with artifacts, scanning the same area from another position will correct the problem.[19, 20]

141. C. Because of the multiple element-sequential firing design of linear-array transducers, the chances for mirror image artifacts are increased.[20]

142. B. The sonographic findings showed both kidneys to be normal in size. However, anechoic areas were seen in both right and left renal sinus and pelvis. These patterns were centrally located (with good through transmission and acoustic enhancement) and consistent with bilateral hydronephrosis. The bladder was not well distended, and the bladder wall appeared markedly thickened, measuring 13 mm. The prostate appeared heterogeneous with both hypoechoic areas and hyperechoic areas. There was a discrete hyperechoic area (35 × 29 mm) protruding into the urinary bladder that appeared contiguous with the prostate. The prostate was enlarged and measured 47 × 42 × 48 mm excluding the hyperechoic area. On the basis of these films, the diagnostic impression and differential diagnosis were benign prostatic hypertrophy (BPH). Prostatic carcinoma and bladder neoplasm could not be ruled out.

143. B. The bladder wall is normally seen on sonography as a thin, smooth, echogenic interface that varies in thickness depending on the degree of bladder distention. Some experts consider the bladder wall enlarged if it measures greater than 5 mm,[28] while others consider the bladder wall to be within normal limits when it measures between 3 to 6 mm.[11]

144. A. Visualization of the liver and kidney was enhanced by the abnormal presence of a large amount of ascitic fluid.

145. C. Hemangiomas are frequently seen in women and patients of advancing age. Histologically, hemangiomas are arteriovenous malformations composed of vascular endothelium lined spaces filled with red blood cells. These lesions are most commonly located in the posterior right liver lobe.[17]

146. D. The typical ultrasound appearance of a hemangioma is that of a densely echogenic, homogeneous mass with sharply marginated borders.[17]

147. D. Septated cysts were seen in both the right and left liver lobes. The measurements of the right-lobe cyst was approximately 12.3 × 8.7 × 12.4 cm in anterior-posterior and transverse dimension. The gallbladder, common duct, pancreas, and kidney were seen in additional scans and appeared normal. Correlation with liver CT scan was suggested. Smooth borders are usual in cysts. Sonographically,

cysts appear sonolucent with posterior enhancement and sharp, well-defined borders. A patient with a liver cyst is usually asymptomatic unless a large cyst interferes with liver function. Normally the cysts are small and found incidentally. If the walls are irregular and through transmission is variable, the cyst may be aspirated; otherwise, nothing is done.[8] (Courtesy of Joanne Cramer, Johns Hopkins School of Ultrasound, Baltimore, MD.)

148. D. The ultrasound report indicated the presence of marked retroperitoneal lymphadenopathy. CT scans of the abdomen and pelvis confirmed the ultrasound findings.

149. D. The ultrasound findings were consistent with the presence of a small angiomyolipoma. A HIDA scan was performed and was negative for acute cholecystitis. No other studies were performed. Isolated angiomyolipomas are most commonly found in females age 40 to 50 years. Diagnostic confirmation of the diagnosis of angiomyolipoma is usually made when computed tomography (CT) reveals the presence of fat within this type of mass.[19]

150. C. Wilms' tumor most often presents as a palpable mass, but may cause nonspecific symptoms such as pain, fever, malaise, and weight loss. The peak age is 3 to 4 years, but adult and infant cases have been detected on sonography as solid masses arising from the area of the renal sinus, displacing and distorting the kidney.[11]

151. A. Wilms' tumors may appear complex and contain anechoic or cystic spaces, which probably represent necrosis or hemorrhage.[11]

152. C. Ultrasound of the abdomen indicated hepatosplenomegaly with extensive hepatic metastatic disease. Dilatation of the intrahepatic radicles, gallbladder, and CBD were noted, indicating extrahepatic biliary obstruction. The cause of the obstruction could not be demonstrated. The left kidney was found to measure only 7 cm, consistent with chronic renal parenchymal disease. No additional studies were performed to confirm the ultrasound findings.

153. B. The presence of the dilated ureter extending from the renal pelvis indicates that the obstruction is not at the ureteropelvic junction.[20]

154. D. The most common kidney function tests are blood urea nitrogen (BUN), serum creatinine level, and creatinine clearance. It is impor-

tant for sonographers to understand that BUN measures the concentration of nitrogen as urea in the blood (formed largely through
protein metabolism), and that creatinine is primarily a by-product
of muscle metabolism. Values for both tests are elevated if reduced
filtration is present. Creatinine clearance is the amount of blood
theoretically "cleared" of creatinine in 1 minute by filtration. If renal filtration is impaired, creatinine clearance decreases, since less
blood is cleared of creatinine by the kidney.[5]

155. C. This case was felt to represent the presence of a focal thrombus
in the upper aspect of the IVC. It was believed to be chronic due to
its marked echogenicity and possibly occurred secondary to the
prior use of an indwelling catheter. According to Sauerbrie et al.,
benign thrombus inside the IVC is usually due to extension of the
thrombus from the iliac veins or renal veins. In neonates and infants, causes include indwelling catheters (umbilical vein catheters), dehydration, and sepsis. The thrombus, which may partially
or completely fill the lumen and distend the IVC, usually demonstrates low- to mid-level echoes. Calcification may occur in cases of
long-standing thrombus.[22]

156. C. Nephrocalcinosis is the deposit of calcium within the kidney
parenchyma. Both kidneys are usually affected with nephrocalcinosis and the condition exists as either cortical nephrocalcinosis or
medullary nephrocalcinosis. With cortical nephrocalcinosis focal or
diffuse, punctate or confluent densities appear within the cortex of
the kidney creating a dense kidney outline. No acoustic shadowing
is present. With medullary nephrocalcinosis the cortical echoes are
normal but focal areas of increased echogenicity are found in the
area of the renal pyramids. There is no acoustic shadowing associated with these densities because the calculi are too small to cast
shadows. This condition can occur in children with hyper-
parathyroidism, renal tubular acidosis, hypercalcemia, and particularly those infants receiving long-term furosemide or lasix for
chronic lung or heart disease.[11,21]

157. B. Pyloric stenosis involves the enlargement of the pyloric muscle,
the channel between the stomach and the duodenum. Affected children present with vomiting between ages 1 week and 6 months,
and ultrasound (the examination of choice) should employ trans-
verse/oblique scans that follow the lesser curvature of the stomach
through the left liver lobe, just to the right of the midline. The antrum of the stomach lies anterior and left of the lumbar spine (in
transverse plane) and the pylorus is continuous with the stomach.

In pyloric stenosis, the pyloric diameter should be 1.5 cm or greater, its muscle length should be 2 cm or greater, and thickness at least 4 mm.[11]

158. A. Hypertrophic pyloric stenosis presents a doughnut sign: an anechoic to hypoechoic muscle mass with a central lumen of increased echogenicity reflecting from the mucosa. Measurements should be made from the antrum of the stomach to the most distal portion of the identifiable channel. If the tumor or pylorus is not well-visualized, the patient may drink some water to display the gastric lumen.[11]

159. C. Reidel's lobe is a normal variant in which the right lobe of the liver extends past the right kidney anteriorly, sometimes reaching even to the iliac crest.[2]

160. C. The thin, tongue-like projection of the right lobe of the liver can give the false impression of hepatomegaly. However, since Reidel's lobe is a normal variant it would be helpful to scan the left lobe of the liver, which is typically very small in such patients.[2]

REFERENCES

1. Burke SR. Human anatomy and physiology for the health sciences. New York: John Wiley & Sons, 1980.

2. Buurma G. Guidelines for abdomen review. Dallas: Society of Diagnostic Medical Sonographers, 1991.

3. Chen J-J, Changchien C-S, Chiou S-S, et al. Various sonographic patterns of smooth muscle tumors of the gastrointestinal tract. J Ultrasound Med 1992;11:527.

4. Craig M. Pocket guide to ultrasound measurements. Philadelphia: JB Lippincott, 1987.

5. Ferguson GG. Pathophysiology: mechanisms and expressions. Philadelphia: WB Saunders, 1984.

6. Govan ADT, Macfarlane PS, Callander R. Pathology illustrated. Edinburgh: Churchill Livingstone, 1981.

7. Hagen-Ansert SL. The anatomy workbook. Philadelphia: JB Lippincott, 1986.

8. Hagen-Ansert SL. Textbook of diagnostic ultrasonography. 3rd ed. St Louis: CV Mosby, 1989.

9. Hall R. The ultrasound handbook. Philadelphia: JB Lippincott, 1988.

10. Huang Y-S, Lee S-D, Wu J-C, Wang S-S, Lin H-C, Tsai Y-T. Utility of sonographic gallbladder wall patterns in differentiating malignant from cirrhotic ascites. J Clin Ultrasound 1989;17:187.

11. Kawamura D. Diagnostic medical sonography. Vol III: Abdomen. Philadelphia: JB Lippincott, 1992.

12. Kremkau FW. Diagnostic ultrasound: principles, instruments, and exercises. 3rd ed. Philadelphia, WB Saunders, 1989.

13. Lanius K, Pearson J. A review of polycystic kidney disease. J Diag Med Sonog 1992;8:232.

14. Lewis E. Screening for diffuse and focal liver disease. J Clin Ultrasound 1984;12:67.

15. Lin Z-Y, Chang W-Y, Wang L-Y, et al. Duplex pulsed doppler sonography of hepatocellular carcinoma treated with transcatheter arterial embolization. J Ultrasound Med 1991;10:619.

16. Metreweli C. Practical abdominal ultrasound. Chicago: Year Book Medical Publishers, 1978.

17. Mittelstaedt CA. Abdominal ultrasound. New York: Churchill Livingstone, 1987.

18. Pansky B. Dynamic anatomy and physiology. New York: Macmillan, 1975.

19. Rumack CM, Wilson ST, Charboneau WJ. Diagnostic ultrasound. Vol II. St. Louis: Mosby Year Book, 1991.

20. Sanders RC. Clinical sonography: a practical approach. Boston: Little Brown, 1983.

21. Sarti DA. Diagnostic ultrasound text and cases. 2nd ed. Chicago: Year Book Medical Publishers, 1987.

22. Sauerbrei EE, Nguyen KT, Nolan RL. Abdominal sonography. New York: Raven Press, 1992.

23. Shimamoto K, Sakuma S, Ishigaki T, et al. Hepatocellular carcinoma: evaluation with color Doppler ultrasound and MR imaging. Radiology 1992;182:149.

24. Teefey SA, Baron RL, Radke HM, et al. Gangrenous cholecystitis: new observations on sonography. J Ultrasound Med 1991;10:603.

25. Teele R, Share JC. Ultrasonography of infants and children. Philadelphia: WB Saunders, 1991.

26. Towers MJ, Withers CE, Rachlis AR, et al. Ultrasound diagnosis of hepatic Kaposi's sarcoma. J Ultrasound Med 1991;10:701.

Marveen Craig: *Ultrasound Exam Review*, © 1994 J. B. Lippincott Co.

3

Superficial Structures

OBJECTIVES

High-resolution ultrasound systems have improved the imaging of shallow anatomy to such an extent that they now enable dramatic visualization of anatomy and pathology at depths of approximately 2 to 5 cm. The operation of such equipment tests the sonographer's acquired and experiential knowledge by demanding skillful use of the optimum focal zone, improvisation of techniques to fit specific patients, and recognition of technical artifacts and deceptive pathology. This chapter is designed to test your knowledge of a variety of applications in what, to many, are sometimes less familiar studies.

QUESTIONS

Directions
Each of the questions or incomplete statements is followed by several answers or completions. Select the best answer(s) in each case. In the matching sections, answers should be used only once, unless otherwise stated.

1. Hematomas of the abdominal wall musculature are easily imaged with ultrasound. Which of the following conditions is (are) most likely to be associated with the development of such hematomas?
   A. Trauma; collagen disorders
   B. Debilitating diseases; infections
   C. Pregnancy; puerperium
   D. All of the above

2. Hashimoto's disease can also be described as:
   A. granulomatosis.
   B. lymphadenoid goiter.
   C. subacute thyroiditis.
   D. giant cell thyroiditis.

3. Hydroceles are most commonly seen in:
   A. newborns.
   B. men between the ages of 15–30.
   C. men over 60.
   D. boys between the ages of 7–12.

4. Pitfalls involving the sonographic evaluation of a Baker's cyst include:
   A. hyperextension of the leg.
   B. artifacts.
   C. popliteal artery aneurysm or other inflammatory processes.
   D. all of the above

5. A 33-year-old male was referred from his urologist for scrotal sonography. His chief complaint was of a "dull ache" in the left testicle. Physical examination and transillumination confirmed the presence of a complex, primarily solid mass enveloping the testis. Anechoic and septated areas were interspersed among the normal parenchyma. Lab studies were obtained and revealed elevation of AFP and HCG. The patient went to surgery. The findings in this case are highly suggestive of:
   A. seminoma.
   B. varicocele.
   C. choriocarcinoma.
   D. sarcoma.

6. Which of the following transducer frequencies is best for evaluating an abdominal aortic aneurysm graft?
   A. 3.5–5 MHz
   B. 5–7.5 MHz
   C. 10 MHz
   D. 20 MHz

7. Sonography of the chest is generally performed with patients in the:
   A. supine position with arms elevated.
   B. upright position with arms outstretched.
   C. sitting up and inclined forward onto or over a support.
   D. on either side (decubitus).

8. Sonography is of diagnostic value in the IV drug user who suffers complications secondary to various mixing agents and injection techniques. Venous sclerosis forces such patients to use larger, more central veins. Two popular locations to investigate for the presence of abscesses, hematomas, venous occlusion, or thrombosis are the:
    A. feet and thighs.
    B. groin and neck.
    C. hands and axilla.
    D. all of the above

9. A scrotal hernia containing omentum or other fatty masses will appear:
    A. isoechoic.
    B. anechoic.
    C. to present high amplitude echoes.
    D. heterogeneous.

10. Sonographic findings in thyroid adenomas include the following:
    A. a peripheral "halo."
    B. an homogeneous echogenicity of lower magnitude than normal thyroid tissue.
    C. an heterogeneous echogenicity of greater magnitude than normal thyroid tissue.
    D. A and B

11. In epididymitis, color-flow Doppler should demonstrate _____ to the area.
    A. decreased blood flow
    B. increased blood flow
    C. turbulent blood flow
    D. no flow

12. The development of benign breast cysts in postmenopausal females is associated with:
    A. estrogen therapy.
    B. hypertension medications.
    C. steroids, digitalis.
    D. all of the above

13. In the context of superficial scanning the terms *Spigelian*, *epigastric, femoral*, and *inguinal* all refer to:
    A. obstructions.
    B. aneurysms.
    C. hernias.
    D. tumors.

14. The ultrasound diagnosis of varicocele depends on the visualization of an increased number and size of scrotal veins. Duplex Doppler is critical in such cases to assess:
    A. venous flow and competency.
    B. incompetent valves.
    C. thrombosis, hematoma.
    D. A and B

15. Technical aid(s) to improved thyroid scanning is (are):
    A. coronal scans with the patient in the decubitus position.
    B. hyperextending the patient's neck.
    C. observation during swallowing.
    D. B and C

16. Inflammatory urachal cysts may spontaneously drain into the:
    A. urinary bladder.
    B. umbilicus.

C. rectum.

D. A and B

17. Which of the following statements about aortic aneurysms is (are) *inaccurate?*
    A. Diameters >3 cm are considered aneurysmal
    B. Mycotic aneurysms are the result of trauma
    C. Male predominance; rare before 50 years of age
    D. Pseudoaneurysms best evaluated with Doppler

18. Identify the numbered structures shown in Figure 3-1.

    1. ___   A. Prostate gland
    2. ___   B. Corpus cavernosum of the penis
    3. ___   C. Corpus spongiosum of the penis
    4. ___   D. Seminal vesicle
    5. ___   E. Rectum
    6. ___   F. Testis
    7. ___   G. Ductus deferens

    8. ___   H. Urinary bladder
    9. ___   I. Urethra
    10. ___   J. Epididymis

19. Which of the following statements about graded compression sonography is (are) *untrue?*
    A. It is particularly helpful in cases of acute appendicitis
    B. It eliminates overlying bowel gas and fluid to improve visualization of the appendix
    C. It will not compress an inflamed, obstructed appendix
    D. It should be applied gradually starting in the midline and moving to the right

20. Which of the following statements are characteristic of aortic aneurysms?
    A. Rupture rate greatest >5 cm
    B. Diffuse enlargement denotes a saccular aneurysm
    C. Atherosclerosis is a causative factor
    D. A and C

21. With state-of-the-art equipment it is possible to detect breast tumors _____ in size.
    A. 3 cm
    B. 2 cm
    C. >1 cm
    D. <1 cm

22. Retroperitoneal fibrosis associated with abdominal aortic aneurysms is also referred to as a (an):
    A. inflammatory aneurysm.

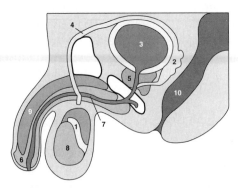

Figure 3-1. Sagittal view of the male pelvis.

B. mycotic aneurysm.

C. pseudoaneurysm.

D. laminated aneurysm.

23. Spermatoceles are frequently encountered and usually occur in the:
    A. testes.
    B. epididymis.
    C. seminal vesicles.
    D. pampiniform plexus.

24. Scrotal wall thickness is normally:
    A. 2–3 mm.
    B. 2–4 mm.
    C. 2–6 mm.
    D. 2–8 mm.

25. The presence of an enlarged testis within the inguinal canal in males aged 5 and above raises the concern of:
    A. concomitant pathology.
    B. ischemia.
    C. infection.
    D. intussusception.

26. In patients with laboratory findings of hypercalcemia and hypophosphatemia, what organ(s) should be scanned?
    A. Aorta and kidneys
    B. Parathyroid
    C. Liver
    D. Carotid arteries

27. Which of the following statements concerning rotator cuff scanning is (are) *inaccurate?*
    A. Frequencies of 7 MHz or higher should be used
    B. Transducer of choice is the linear-array
    C. Transducer should be maintained perpendicular to the tendon
    D. The bicipital groove in the proximal humerus should be used as a reference landmark

28. A 65-year-old female (G4P4) was referred to the ultrasound department with a 12-year history of a large, egg-shaped mass in the lower outer quadrant of the right breast. Palpation of the mass revealed it to be smooth, hard, and mobile. Breast sonography demonstrated a 60 × 50 × 40 mm cystic mass with increased posterior transmission. In the upper corner of the mass an echogenic projection and internal trabeculae were noted. These findings would suggest:
    A. simple cyst.
    B. intracystic papilloma.
    C. adenocarcinoma.
    D. papillotubular carcinoma.

29. In scanning patients with suspected deep venous thrombosis, a finding of pulsatile venous flow is suggestive of:
    A. fluid overload and congestive heart failure.
    B. tricuspid insufficiency.
    C. lymphadenopathy or thrombus.
    D. A and B

30. What other sites are most likely to be involved with breast cancer?
    A. Endometrium and ovaries
    B. Colon
    C. Contralateral breast
    D. All of the above

31. Sonographic examination of the spinal cord is possible in infants under 6 months of age because of incomplete ossification of the posterior spinous processes. Among the observations that can be made are:
    A. cord pulsations and movements.
    B. cauda equina.
    C. central end of the median fissure.
    D. all of the above

32. A normal variant of the thyroid gland is the _____ lobe.
    A. semilunar
    B. pyramidal
    C. thymal
    D. sinister

33. It is important to evaluate the _____ in patients who have iliac artery aneurysms.
    A. kidneys
    B. pancreas
    C. mesentery
    D. adrenals

34. Which of the following statements about ultrasound-assisted biopsy is (are) untrue?
    A. Needles must traverse the scanning plane
    B. Noncoated needles are generally easier to identify than Teflon-coated needles
    C. Biopsy guides attached to the transducer simplify the procedure
    D. Biopsy procedures should be continuously monitored with ultrasound

35. A 45-year-old, unmarried female was referred for breast ultrasound. At the age of 25, the patient noted a small, dense, mobile mass at the outer upper quadrant of her breast, but did not consult a doctor. Recent sonography revealed the presence of a 45 × 45 × 25 mm oval mass containing fine, homogeneous internal echoes. The boundaries of the mass were well defined and the posterior mass border was well accentuated. The most likely finding is:
    A. lipoma.
    B. scirrhous carcinoma.
    C. fibroadenoma.
    D. papilloma.

36. Although the majority of aortic aneurysms occurs in the distal aorta, it is critically important that sonographers demonstrate the relationship of any possible aneurysms in the following arteries:
    A. popliteal and iliac.
    B. renal.
    C. celiac axis.
    D. all of the above

37. Which of the following statements about thyroid function is untrue?
    A. Insufficiency of thyroid hormone in the infant is consistent with cretinism
    B. Hyposecretion of thyroid hormones causes an increase in the BMR (basal metabolic rate)
    C. Severe hypothyroidism can lead to psychiatric symptoms
    D. Thyrotoxicosis is associated with Grave's disease

38. Abdominal wall hernias consist of a:

A. neck, body, tail.
B. sac, contents, covering.
C. muscle, bowel, peritoneum.
D. fat, mucous membrane, subcutaneous tissue.

39. The development of an echogenic band surrounding a testicular neoplasm is associated with the presence of a (an):
A. Sertoli-Leydig tumor.
B. arrhenoblastoma.
C. seminoma.
D. embryonal cell carcinoma.

40. Sonographic findings associated with a full-thickness tear of the rotator cuff include all of the following *except:*
A. joint effusion and absence of normal tendons.
B. elevation of the humeral surface.
C. change in tendon echogenicity.
D. concavity of the supraspinous tendon.

41. The normal size of the adult testicle is _____ cm in length and _____ cm in width and AP diameter.
A. 3–5; 2–3
B. 2–4; 1–2
C. 4–5; 4–6
D. 6–8; 5–7

42. Identify the numbered structures shown in Figure 3-2.

1. ___   A. Cooper's ligament
2. ___   B. Retromammary layer
3. ___   C. Pectoralis major
4. ___   D. Subcutaneous fat

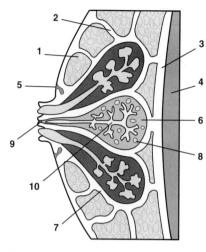

Figure 3-2. Cross-sectional diagram of the female breast.

5. ___   E. Acinus
6. ___   F. Ampulla
7. ___   G. Interlobular connective tissues
8. ___   H. Superficial fascia
9. ___   I. Montgomery's gland
10. ___   J. Lactiferous duct

43. Sonography of the chest is valuable in demonstrating which of the following?
A. Atelectasis and pleural thickening
B. Evaluation of the diaphragm and pleural effusion
C. Thoracic masses, empyema and hemothorax
D. All of the above

44. Which of the following is (are) *not* accurate statements concerning the abdominal aorta?
A. Aortic grafts will not pulsate

B. Aortic dilatation in excess of 3 cm is considered aneurysmal

C. A saccular aneurysm is one in which the aorta weaves from side to side

D. All of the above

45. Nonspecific epididymitis with subsequent orchitis is usually the result of:

A. trauma.

B. gonorrhea.

C. urinary tract infections.

D. chlamydial infections.

46. The thyroid responds to iodine hunger by:

A. enlarging.

B. developing fatty infiltrates.

C. adding new cells.

D. all of the above

47. Which of the following statements concerning the epididymis is *untrue*?

A. Conveys sperm from testes to seminal vesicles

B. Are divided into two parts: head and body

C. Head may appear crescent-shaped on transverse views

D. Normally 7–11 mm in size

48. Ultrasound is a valuable tool in the diagnosis of congenital hip displacement. The appearance of the hip socket in cases of dysplasia is characteristically:

A. concave, deeper than normal.

B. flat and shallower than normal.

C. convex and shallow.

D. irregular and rough.

49. Rupture is rare in peripheral aneurysms such as the popliteal, femoral, and subclavian arteries. However, because of the common threats of _____, ultrasound—especially Doppler ultrasound—plays a key diagnostic role.

A. lumenal thrombosis and distal embolization

B. tortuosity

C. sluggish flow

D. all of the above

50. Identify the numbered anatomical structures shown in Figure 3-3.

1. ___   A. Bulbous corpus cavernosum

2. ___   B. Testis

3. ___   C. Ejaculatory duct

4. ___   D. Urinary bladder

5. ___   E. Corpus cavernosum penis

6. ___   F. Prostate

7. ___   G. Epididymis

8. ___   H. Urethra

9. ___   I. Scrotum

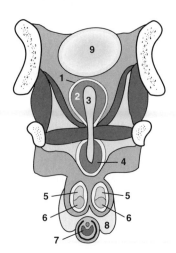

Figure 3-3. Coronal section of male pelvis.

51. Acute scrotal pain is a frequent complaint in adult males. The primary clinical concern is:
    A. epididymitis.
    B. testicular ischemia.
    C. hemorrhagic trauma.
    D. A and C

52. During thyroid scanning it is possible to observe the following muscle group(s):
    A. longus colli.
    B. strap.
    C. sternocleidomastoid.
    D. all of the above

53. During examination of a patient with pleural effusion, it is important to obtain images in (on):
    A. inspiration and expiration and both right and left sides.
    B. both supine and upright positions.
    C. the same position the patient will assume during actual biopsy.
    D. both right and left lateral decubitus positions.

54. High-frequency real-time imaging is indicated for breast scanning. The optimal transducer frequency is:
    A. 3.5 MHz.
    B. 5 MHz.
    C. 7.5 MHz.
    D. B and C

55. There are three basic types of aortic aneurysms: fusiform, saccular, and dissecting. The dissecting aneurysm is usually found in the _____, while the fusiform aneurysm is usually found in the _____.
    A. abdominal aorta; thoracic aorta
    B. thoracic aorta; abdominal aorta
    C. anywhere along the aorta
    D. at the aortic bifurcation

56. Which of the following statements about endemic goiters is *untrue?*
    A. Caused by dietary insufficiency of iodine
    B. More frequent in males than females
    C. More common during puberty
    D. Generally do not attain the size of multinodular goiters

57. Use the following anatomical terms to label the numbered structures in Figure 3-4.

    1. _____   A. Longus colli muscle
    2. _____   B. Trachea
    3. _____   C. Jugular vein

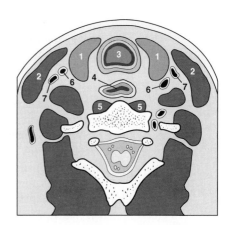

Figure 3-4. Thyroid and neck anatomy.

4. ___ D. Sternocleido-
        mastoid muscle
5. ___ E. Esophagus
6. ___ F. Carotid artery
7. ___ G. Thyroid

58. The sonographic appearance of a urachal cyst is that of a tubular, echo-free structure located in the:
    A. pelvis.
    B. upper abdomen.
    C. lower abdominal wall.
    D. iliac fossa.

59. Which of the following statements concerning the appendix is *untrue*?
    A. Originates at the tip of the cecum
    B. Ends in a blind pouch
    C. Demonstrates peristalsis
    D. May become inflamed or obstructed

60. Real-time examination of the parathyroid gland should be concentrated in the area extending from the _____, to the superior aspect of the thyroid gland, and laterally to the _____.
    A. superior sternal notch; sternocleidomastoid muscles
    B. superior pole of the clavicle; carotid and jugular vessels
    C. mid-portion of the hyoid cartilage; carotid artery
    D. mid-portion of the sternal notch; jugular vein

61. During a survey of the scrotum, scans of the _____ should be made with the patient engaged in quiet respirations and performing a Valsalva maneuver.
    A. bladder
    B. pelvis
    C. spermatic cord
    D. testes

62. Which of the following conditions can be confused with an abdominal aortic aneurysm?
    A. Pancreatic gland or horseshoe kidney
    B. Periaortic nodes
    C. Refraction artifacts
    D. All of the above

63. Differentiation between varicoceles and spermatoceles can be enhanced by:
    A. upright scanning.
    B. color-flow Doppler.
    C. Valsalva maneuver.
    D. all of the above

64. The sonographic demonstration of a thin, linear, mobile echo flap within the arterial lumen is characteristic of:
    A. aortic rupture.
    B. aortic dissection.
    C. aortic graft.
    D. aortic reverberation artifact.

65. The presence of _____ is considered a surgical emergency.
    A. testicular torsion
    B. epididymitis
    C. abscess
    D. all of the above

66. Cryptorchidism is the medical term describing a (an):
    A. congenital anomaly of the tunica albugenia.
    B. atrophy of the rete testes.
    C. undescended testicle.
    D. atresia of the vas deferens.

CASES AND QUESTIONS

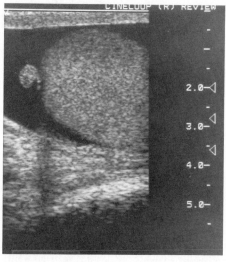 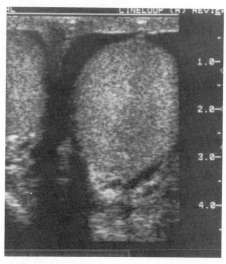

A   *B*

Figure 3-5. (*A*) Longitudinal scan of left testis. (*B*) Transverse scans of left and right testes. (Courtesy of Dayna Lundru & Tracy Pfizenmaier, St. Francis Hospital, Milwaukee, Wisconsin.)

The patient was a 27-year-old male who presented with left testicular swelling.

67. The echogenic protuberance seen superior in the testis in Figure 3-5*A* most likely represents:
    A. malignant tumor.
    B. the mediastinum of the testis.
    C. appendix testis.
    D. testicular torsion.

68. The fluid collection seen in both scans most likely represents a:
    A. hydrocele.
    B. pyocele.
    C. spermatocele.
    D. hematocele.

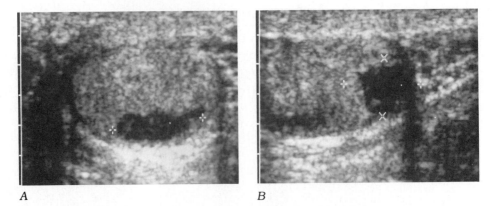

A   *B*

Figure 3-6. (*A*) Transverse scan of the left testis. (*B*) Sagittal scan of the left testis. (Courtesy of Kris Kuros, Rhode Island Hospital School of Diagnostic Medical Sonography, Providence, Rhode Island.)

The patient is a 33-year-old male complaining of an acute onset of intense pain of the left scrotum with swelling and tenderness. Real time and color-flow Doppler scans of the scrotum were ordered to answer the clinical question of abscess collection vs. hematoma or malignant tumor. Doppler revealed increased blood flow to the testis.

69. Both the long and short axis scans presented as Figure 3-6*A* and *B* demonstrate an area of abnormality. The best term(s) to describe that area are:
    A. hyperechoic.
    B. anechoic.
    C. hypoechoic.
    D. isoechoic.

70. This case most likely demonstrates _____ of the left testis.
    A. epididymitis
    B. orchitis
    C. hydrocele
    D. intratesticular tumor

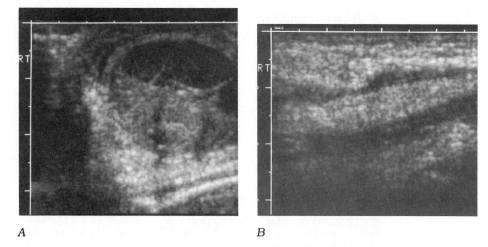

A   *B*

Figure 3-7. (*A*) Transverse scan of the right testis. (*B*) Sagittal scan in the region of the right inguinal canal and right hemiscrotum. (Courtesy of Kathy Toledo, Rhode Island Hospital School of Diagnostic Medical Sonography, Providence, Rhode Island.)

The patient, a 5-year-old male, was admitted for right inguinal exploration after being kicked in the groin while playing. The patient complains of swelling, pain in the right hemiscrotum, dysuria, and tenderness to the right testis and inguinal region.

71. In Figure 3-7*A*, the testis appears normal; however, additional findings are of:
    A. fluid.
    B. debris.
    C. septa.
    D. all of the above

72. The presence of these structures are highly suggestive of:
    A. hydrocele.
    B. hematocele.
    C. abscess.
    D. infarct.

73. In Figure 3-7*B*, what is the significance of the echogenic, nonperistalsing structure within the inguinal canal?
    A. Mesentery, lymph nodes
    B. Omentum, hernia
    C. Lymph nodes
    D. Inguinal ligament

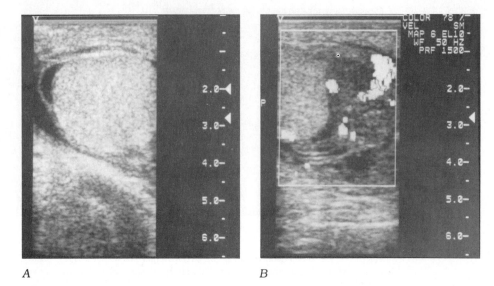

A   B

Figure 3-8. (A) Transverse scan of the left testis. (B) Sagittal scan of the left testis. (Courtesy of Judy Schwartz, State University of New York Health Sciences Center, Brooklyn, New York.)

The patient is a 24-year-old male who presented with severe left scrotal pain and swelling. Sonography of the right testis was normal.

74. What finding in this case rules out testicular torsion?
    A. Fluid around the testicle
    B. A swollen epididymis
    C. Doppler evidence of blood flow
    D. A mass in the testicle

75. Considering knowledge of the presence of flow, what finding is suggested by Figure 3-8A, B?
    A. Trauma
    B. Epididymitis
    C. Orchitis
    D. Hematocele

ANSWERS

1. D. Hematomas are generally associated with muscle trauma that results in hemorrhage. They can also result from infection, debilitating disease, collagen disorders, pregnancy, and childbirth. Straining,
   coughing and anticoagulant therapy can also be precipitating
   factors.[13, 18]

2. B. Hashimoto's disease is a chronic inflammatory disease of the
   thyroid. It is also known as chronic thyroiditis and is a progressive
   disease that most frequently affects women 10 to 50 years of age. It
   is thought to be autoimmune. Subacute thyroiditis, granulomatosis, and giant cell thyroiditis are one and the same. They describe
   an inflammatory condition of probable viral origin.[3, 4, 9, 13]

3. A. Hydroceles, the most common fluid collection of the scrotum, occur in both children and adults. Hydrocele is most common in newborns (congenital hydrocele), since the processus vaginalis, which
   connects the scrotal sac with the peritoneum, is still open.[13] (Courtesy of Dayna Lundru and Tracy Pfizenmaier, St. Francis School of
   Diagnostic Medical Sonography, Milwaukee, Wisconsin.)

4. D. A Baker's cyst is a fluid-filled collection posterior to the knee
   joint caused by the escape of synovial fluid which becomes enclosed
   in a sac of membranous tissue. Usually occurring laterally, it may
   cause swelling resulting from compression of the popliteal vein and
   associated venous drainage.[30] Undue extension of the leg will
   obliterate a Baker's cyst that communicates with the knee joint because the fluid will return into the knee joint proper.[24] Purulent in-
   flammations of adjacent cellular tissue or popliteal artery
   aneurysms may have a similar sonographic appearance. Scanning
   with lower frequency transducers can produce confusing reverberation artifacts that may obscure pathology.

5. C. Choriocarcinoma is a rare germ-cell tumor. Serum markers of
   HCG (human chorionic gonadotrophin) and AFP (alpha fetoprotein)
   are elevated in the presence of mixed germ-cell tumors and non-
   seminomatous tumors.[3, 11, 13]

6. B. Because of their relatively superficial location, grafts are best
   evaluated with a transducer frequency of 5 MHz or greater.[10] Aortic
   grafts are usually man-made tubular structures used to repair an
   aortic aneurysm. The grafted replacements are easily detected by a
   characteristic wall brightness, and at times it is also possible to see
   their ribbing.[1] Graft walls can be recognized by the presence of lin-

ear parallel echoes within the host vessel.[24] New fluid collections around or adjacent to a graft may be due to hematoma, seroma, or abscess.[8] Higher-frequency transducers are preferred to identify and distinguish between the echo patterns of organizing clot, viscous pus, etc., and reverberation. Color Doppler ultrasound or pulsed wave Doppler are extremely valuable in differentiating between true and false (pseudo) aneurysms and in suspected graft occlusion.[26]

7. C. Ultrasound of the chest is best performed with the patient in a sitting position. The patient may straddle a chair and lean against a pillow placed on the chair back. This will allow the examiner easy access to the back of the patient's chest and will help to stabilize the patient.[3]

8. B. Because an inevitable consequence of frequent injection of foreign substances is peripheral venous sclerosis, the IV drug user is forced to utilize larger, more central veins. Usually the groin ("groin hit") and the neck ("pocket shot") are favored.[16]

9. C. A scrotal hernia presents a sonographic image of the presence of an echogenic, extratesticular mass which contains echogenic and anechoic areas related to the air-fluid contents of loops of bowel that have descended through the inguinal canal.[23, 29] (Courtesy of Kathy Toledo, Rhode Island Hospital School of Diagnostic Medical Sonography, Providence, Rhode Island.)

10. D. The sonographic appearance of thyroid adenoma on ultrasound is homogeneous with echogenicity varying from more to less than that of normal thyroid tissue. Frequently a halo is seen surrounding the periphery of the nodule.[3, 13]

11. B. In patients with epididymitis, color Doppler will show increased blood flow due to tissue hyperemia.[13] (Courtesy of Judy Schwartz, State University of New York Health Science Center, Brooklyn, New York.)

12. D. Cysts, the most common breast lesion, are almost always benign. They are usually associated with a variety of conditions of epithelial origin, collectively termed *fibrocystic disease*. Cysts occur most often in menstruating women between the ages of 35 and 50 years. Generally, they subside after menopause, but postmenopausal women who take estrogen, blood pressure medications, steroids, or digitalis may develop cysts.[13]

13. C. Hernias of the abdominal wall are readily diagnosed by an appropriate history and physical examination. There are, however, a small number of patients, usually obese, who have clinical occult hernias and who present with abdominal pain of unknown origin. Spigelian, epigastric, lumbar, femoral and inguinal hernias can mimic symptoms of renal, biliary, or gastrointestinal diseases.[13, 28]

14. D. Sonographic identification of varicocele depends on the visualization of an increased number and size of scrotal veins. The varicose condition of the veins of the pampiniform plexus are secondary to the phenomenon of incompetent valves in the internal spermatic vein. Duplex Doppler is indicated to assess the competence of the internal spermatic vein and to assess the ultrasound criteria in diagnosing varicoceles.[15, 25]

15. D. Hyperextending the patient's neck over pillows or bolsters provides a more planar scanning surface for direct scanning techniques. Visualizing the lower poles of the thyroid can often be improved by having the patient swallow, which raises the gland superiorly.[24, 30]

16. D. A patent urachus is the result of persistence of the allantoic canal between the bladder and the umbilicus. Urine may drain constantly from the umbilicus. A partially patent urachus means that the urachus communicates with either the umbilicus (urachal sinus) or the bladder. If an inflamed urachal cyst remains untreated, spontaneous drainage into the bladder or umbilicus can result.[13, 19, 26]

17. B. Mycotic aneurysms are the least common type and occur as a result of bacterial infection. Mostly saccular in nature, their common sonographic feature is of asymmetric wall thickening.[3] The abdominal aorta is the most commonly affected artery and is considered aneurysmal whenever it exceeds 3 cm in diameter.[24, 26] Doppler is advantageous in making the diagnosis of pseudoaneurysm versus hematoma by demonstrating blood flow within the mass.[3, 13]

18. 1. J, 2. D, 3. H, 4. G, 5. A, 6. C, 7. I, 8. F, 9. B, 10. E[3, 13]

19. D. When performed by an experienced operator, graded compression sonography may be of considerable clinical value in cases of questionable acute appendicitis. Although normal bowel can readily be compressed with moderate pressure, Puylaert noted that the inflamed obstructed appendix will not compress.[21] The use of com-

pression also eliminates overlying bowel gas and fluid and brings
the appendix within view of a high-resolution transducer (5–7.5
MHz). Compression must be applied to the *right lower quadrant*
very gradually to avoid eliciting peritoneal signs.[12, 21]

20. D. The term *fusiform* correctly describes a diffusely enlarged aneurysm. A saccular aneurysm produces a sac-like protrusion on one
side or the other.[13]

21. D. Although it has repeatedly been claimed that sonography of the
breast is unable to detect early breast carcinoma, the development
of hand-held, linear-array transducers in the 7.5 MHz frequency
range now allows malignant tumors less than 1 cm in diameter to
be visualized and biopsies to be performed under real-time ultrasound guidance.[5]

22. A. The literature refers to retroperitoneal fibrosis associated with
abdominal aortic aneurysms as an inflammatory aneurysm. The
abundant inflammatory cells are found in the dense periaortic
fibrosis that encases the aneurysm. The sonographic feature of
periaortic fibrosis is of an aortic aneurysm with a sonolucent halo—
which may be mistaken for a leaking aortic aneurysm. This knowledge is important because the thick, shiny white fibrotic reaction
prevents aortic resection and grafting in the usual manner.[2]

23. A. A spermatocele is a retention cyst which results from partial obstruction of the efferent ductules of the epididymis. The cyst contains milky fluid composed of sperm and lipids. Spermatoceles
usually occur in the head of the epididymis, but may also occur in
the body or tail.[3, 13, 24]

24. D. The scrotum is a musculocutaneous pouch composed of several
layers of tissue: Dartos tunica, external spermatic fascia, middle
spermatic fascia, cremaster muscle, internal spermatic fascia, and
tunica vaginalis. The thickness of the scrotal wall varies from 2 to
8 mm.[13]

25. A. In the absence of palpable testicles, sonography should be used
as a screening modality. In 70% to 80% of cases the undescended
testicle will be located in the inguinal canal. The sonographic diagnosis of undescended testicle is based on the recognition of a
mass with uniformly distributed medium level echoes. The size of
the mass is extremely important. In the newborn period, it should
equal the size of the opposite descended testis. With age, atrophy of
the undescended testicle will occur. Infertility and an almost 50%

increased chance of developing carcinoma are two serious consequences of this condition. Therefore, at ages 5 and above, normal or enlarged testes within the inguinal canal raise the possibility of concomitant pathology.[13,29]

26. B. The function of the parathyroid gland is to secrete a hormone (parathormone) that regulates calcium metabolism and plasma calcium concentration. Increased parathormone secretions result in hypercalcemia and hypophosphatemia. The majority of such cases are caused by parathyroid adenoma.[4]

27. C. The transducer should be maintained parallel to the tendon imaged, as angled views may cause false echogenicity differences.[14]

28. B. Intracystic papillomas are uncommon lesions that usually affect older women. The papilloma grows from a fibrovascular stalk into the lumen of a serous or hemorrhagic cyst.[11,13]

29. D. Pulsatile venous flow suggests congestive heart failure, fluid overload, or tricuspid insufficiency.[30] Lymphadenopathy sometimes results in a false-positive diagnosis of deep venous thrombosis. Thrombus is associated with sluggish flow.[1]

30. D. Metastases of cancer to the breast from distant sites is uncommon but can include cancer of the lung, ovary, uterus, colon, malignant lymphoma, or melanoma. The most common site is the contralateral breast. Primary breast cancer can metastasize to distant organs such as the nodes, liver, lung, and brain, as well as bone.[11,22] (Courtesy of Cathy Shupe, Orange Coast College, Costa Mesa, California.)

31. D. Sonographic imaging of the neonatal spine can demonstrate the normal movements and pulsations of the cord within the spinal canal. In transverse views a bright echogenic dot can be seen in the center of the cord. Originally thought to represent the central canal, it actually represents the central extent of the median fissure. At the caudal end of the spine the cord tapers to form the conus. At the tip of the conus the nerve fibers that make up the cauda equina can be observed as long, thin filaments.[31]

32. B. The pyramidal lobe is a triangular-shaped, superior extension of the isthmus of the thyroid. Present in 15% to 30% of all thyroid glands, it is variable in size and extends more often to the left side. The parenchyma bears the same appearance as the remainder of the normal thyroid.[30]

33. A. The kidneys of patients with known iliac artery aneurysms should be scanned to rule out possible hydronephrosis. The ureters cross the iliac arteries and if aneurysmal, may compress the ureters causing an obstruction.[8]

34. B. Larger needles are more easily seen with ultrasound than smaller needles, and Teflon-coated needles are generally easier to visualize than noncoated needles.[3]

35. C. Fibroadenomas are common, benign, solid tumors composed of a proliferation of connective and epithelial tissues. The incidence rate is higher in patients 15 to 40 years of age and in black women. When palpable these masses are nontender, discrete, firm or rubbery, and movable. The sonographic appearance is of a round or oval smooth-walled mass with uniform, low- to medium-level internal echoes. Minimal to no attenuation or mild enhancement is seen.[3, 13]

36. D. The primary role of sonography in assessing aneurysms is to determine the proximal and distal extent as well as the maximum measurement of the aneurysm. Some aneurysms of the abdominal aorta may involve the celiac axis and the superior mesenteric, renal, and iliac arteries. Special efforts to image these vessels must be made, because surgical management is altered if there is such involvement. Whenever patients with low-placed abdominal aneurysms complain of tingling or numbness in their lower extremities, the popliteal arteries should be examined for possible associated aneurysms.[3, 8, 13, 24]

37. B. Hypothyroidism is the most common disorder affecting the thyroid gland. In children the effects are more devastating than in adults and lead to retarded physical and mental development, called cretinism. Heart rate and body temperature (BMR) are decreased, and there is a tendency toward weight gain. Excess thyroid activity (thyrotoxicosis) can produce Grave's Disease, which occurs primarily in women 20 to 40 years old. One of the dramatic signs of Grave's disease is the development of exophthalmos.[4]

38. B. Abdominal wall hernias consist of three parts: the sac, its contents, and its covering. Hernial contents may consist of any structure in the abdominal cavity and may vary from small pieces of omentum to portions of the bowel.[13]

39. C. On sonography a seminoma appears as a mass with a hypo-echoic homogeneous pattern that may contain scattered hyper-

echoic areas. Seminomas often have a pseudocapsule, which is demonstrated sonographically as an echogenic band surrounding the neoplasm. Most of the testis can be replaced by seminomas, and a reactive hydrocele may be associated.[13]

40. C. A full-thickness rotator cuff tear appears sonographically as an absence of normal tendons. Secondary findings often associated with cuff tears include joint effusion, elevation of humeral surfaces relative to the acromion, irregularity of the humeral joint surfaces, and concavity of the superior margin of the supraspinatus tendon. Diffuse changes in tendon echogenicity suggest inflammation within the cuff, but are *unreliable* indicators of full thickness cuff tears.[14]

41. A. The normal size of adult testicles is 3 to 5 cm in length and 2 to 3 cm in both width and antero-posterior diameters. The testes normally shrink somewhat with age.[13]

42. 1. D, 2. A, 3. B, 4. C, 5. I, 6. G, 7. H, 8. E, 9. F, 10. J[3, 13]

43. D. Pulmonary consolidation or atelectasis appears as an irregular collection of dense echoes arising just beneath the chest wall and extending for a variable depth, depending on the amount of disease. Pleural thickening is manifest by an irregularly thickened echogenic stripe paralleling the chest wall that displaces the lung from the chest wall. Diaphragmatic mobility can be evaluated by observing the diaphragm during deep inspiration and deep expiration. Pleural fluid is easily recognizable as an echo-free space superior to the diaphragm, and posterior and inferior to the lungs. Hemothorax and empyema are suspected when demonstration of a complex but primarily fluid-filled space is seen between the chest wall and the normally aerated lung. The internal echoes may represent an organizing blood clot in the case of hemothorax, or debris in an empyema. Thoracic masses are predominantly echogenic, poorly defined, and transmit sound poorly.[7]

44. C. Aneurysms are pulsatile dilatations of a vessel. In the aorta, the normal diameter at the diaphragm is approximately 2.5 cm; tapering during its inferior course the diameter is approximately 1.5 to 2.0 cm. A true aneurysm is identified sonographically as a dilation of the aorta of 3 cm or greater, near its bifurcation point.[3, 13]

45. C. The most common cause of nonspecific epididymoorchitis is bacterial infection.[11, 23] (Courtesy of Kris Kuros, Rhode Island Hospital School of Diagnostic Medical Sonography, Providence, Rhode Island.)

46. D. The thyroid responds to iodine hunger by growing larger, with the addition of millions of new cells, in an attempt to capture any available iodine. Thyroid weight may shoot up from less than an ounce to several ounces. This condition is known as an iodine-deficient or nontoxic goiter.[3, 13, 19]

47. B. The epididymis store small quantities of sperm prior to ejaculation, convey sperm from the testis to the seminal vesicles, and secrete a small portion of the seminal fluid. They are bilateral and are divided anatomically into three parts: head, body, and tail. Average overall dimensions of the epididymis are $7 \times 11 \times 6$ mm. The normal sonographic appearance of the epididymal head is variable. On longitudinal scans it may have a triangular, crescent, or teardrop shape. The echogenicity of the normal epididymis is homogeneous, equal to or greater than that of the testis, but coarser.[13]

48. B. The diagnosis of congenital hip dysplasia by ultrasound depends on the sonographic demonstration of a hip socket that is characteristically shallow or flat in appearance.[6]

49. A. Color-flow Doppler can measure the size and length of peripheral aneurysms. The presence of lumenal thrombus can be easily identified, with attention given to surface characteristics, noting any irregularities that may give rise to emboli.[27]

50. 1. C, 2. F, 3. H, 4. A, 5. G, 6. B, 7. E, 8. I, 9. D[3, 13]

51. B. Rapid diagnosis of testicular ischemia is critical for preservation of testicular viability, which is optimal up to 12 hours after injury.[24, 26]

52. D. The muscle groups adjacent to the thyroid are the longus colli (posterior); sternocleidomastoid, and strap muscles (anterior and lateral). These hypoechoic muscles are useful when comparing the echogenicity of the thyroid.[10]

53. A. Pleural effusions should be imaged on both inspiration and expiration. When marking a fluid collection for subsequent drainage, it is important to note whether the marking was done in inspiration or expiration. If biopsy or aspiration is not going to be monitored or guided by ultrasound, it is important to conduct the sonography examination in the identical position the patient will assume for the biopsy procedure.[3]

54. D. High-frequency, real-time imaging provides excellent detail of superficial structures and is the most common form of breast so-

nography. Commercially available small-parts transducers operate at frequencies of 5 to 10 MHz and have excellent axial and lateral resolution.[13]

55. B. Dissecting aneurysms occur as a result of a tear in the intimal lining of the vessel. A false lumen is then created within the media of the vessel wall, allowing blood to pass (dissect) between these layers. The intimal flap that is produced appears sonographically as a thin, echogenic linear echo within the lumen of the affected vessel. Motion of the intimal flap in a dissecting aneurysm may be observed with each pulsation. Dissecting aneurysms are most frequently related to systemic hypertension. Other causes are trauma, pregnancy, Marfan's syndrome, congenital bicuspid aortic valve, and aortic isthmus coarctation. Such aneurysms tend to occur in the thoracic portion of the aorta.[3, 13, 24, 26] Fusiform aneurysms present as a tubular swelling of the walls of an artery. Most abdominal aortic aneurysms are fusiform in nature and tend to occur in the distal portion of the abdominal aorta.[3]

56. B. Endemic goiters are more frequently seen in females than in males.[3]

57. 1. G, 2. D, 3. B, 4. E, 5. A, 6. F, 7. C[1, 13]

58. C. The majority of urachal cysts are seen sonographically as anechoic tubular structures in the lower, anterior abdominal wall. Mixed echogenicity, however, may be seen within the cyst when infection is present.[26]

59. C. The appendix originates from the cecal tip, ends in a blind pouch, and has no peristalsis.[20]

60. B. Scanning levels extend from slightly above the sternoclavicular junction (the sternal notch) to the upper-most pole of the thyroid (to include the isthmus). The scans should be extended laterally to include visualization of the carotid artery and jugular vein as reference points.[24]

61. C. Real-time scrotal sonographic evaluation begins with longitudinal oblique scans of the spermatic cord (with both quiet respiration and the Valsalva maneuver to check for varicocele).[13]

62. D. The classic sign of an abdominal aortic aneurysm is the presence of a pulsatile mid-epigastric mass. Transmitted pulsations can occur when the tissues of the pancreas, the horseshoe kidney, or enlarged nodes drape across the aorta, simulating an aneurysm.

Occasionally, transverse scans of the abdomen will produce an apparent duplication of the aorta because of beam refraction at the interface between the rectus abdominis muscles and the collection of fat deep to the linea alba.[13]

63. D. The primary type of varicocele may disappear with the patient in the supine position, so upright scanning may be necessary for its detection. With varicocele, the veins increase in size with abdominal compression, in the erect position, and with the Valsalva maneuver. Secondary varicoceles do not disappear with the patient in the supine position; in this situation the abdomen and pelvis should be scanned carefully to exclude a mass compressing the spermatic vein on the involved side.[13]

64. B. In aortic dissection the intimal lining of the aorta separates from the rest of the wall. Ultrasound demonstrates a thin flap within the aorta that moves with aortic pulsations. There is often an appearance of two lumens: blood flow within the true lumen, and a false lumen created by the space between the dissected intima and the aortic wall. Doppler ultrasound can demonstrate arterial blood flow in both true and false lumens, and it may be impossible to distinguish the two.[13, 26]

65. D. Acute painful scrotum is often a serious presenting symptom. Both epididymitis and torsion can cause severe pain, and it is important to distinguish between the two conditions. Grey-scale ultrasound and color-flow Doppler are the diagnostic tools of choice in distinguishing inflammatory from ischemic processes. Testicular torsion and rupture are surgical emergencies, since in torsion, arterial flow is occluded and only surgical restoration of blood flow can prevent loss of the testicle. Abscess is also an emergency because drainage of the abscess may prevent loss of the testicle. Epididymitis is included in this list because without recognition and treatment, epididymitis may develop into an abscess.[13]

66. C. The term cryptorchidism is used to describe an undescended testicle. Absence of a testicle may be an important finding, since an undescended testicle has 48 times the normal potential for development of cancer.[3, 13]

67. C. The appendix of the testis is found at the upper pole of the testis and is an embryological remnant originally derived from the paramesonephric ducts.[13, 17]

68. A. Inflammation of the testis may cause an accumulation of fluid

within the potential space provided by the two layers of the tunica vaginalis. Such collections are referred to as a *hydrocele*.[3, 13, 17] (Courtesy of Dayna Lundru and Tracy Pfizenmaier, St. Francis School of Diagnostic Medical Sonography, Milwaukee, Wisconsin.)

69. C. Two irregularly hypoechoic lesions appear within the inferior portion of the left testis.

70. B. The sonographic diagnosis was that of orchitis. Orchitis is an infection limited to the testes, which is rare. More frequently, infections occur in the epididymis. Orchitis and epididymitis can be classified as specific (gonorrhea, syphilis, mumps, tuberculosis), nonspecific, and traumatic. In isolated orchitis, increased blood flow would be localized to the testes. It is frequently difficult to assess the epididymal versus testicular nature of this infection because of the difficulty of palpation. With the use of ultrasound it can be determined if testicular involvement is focal or diffuse. Characteristically, focal orchitis produces a hypoechoic area adjacent to an enlarged portion of the epididymis. If left untreated, the entire testicle may become involved, appearing hypoechoic and enlarged. This patient's condition was treated surgically and the pathologic and final diagnoses were that of chronic nongranulomatous orchitis.[11, 23] (Courtesy of Kris Kuros, Rhode Island Hospital School of Diagnostic Ultrasound, Providence, Rhode Island.)

71. D. Surrounding the testis are structures that represent fluid, debris, and septations. These findings are consistent with a hematocele.

72. B. The presence of fluid, debris, and septations are consistent with a hematocele.

73. B. The ultrasound report stated: "The finger-like echogenic structure extending through the internal ring into the canal, down toward the hemiscrotum, were thought to most likely represent omentum, and were thought to be consistent with an incarcerated inguinal hernia. No bowel was seen within the canal or hemiscrotum. Exploratory inguinal hernia repair was carried out and the final diagnosis was that of incarcerated omentum." Scrotal hernias are a common paratesticular mass. Although scrotal hernias are usually diagnosed on the basis of clinical history, sonography is useful in the evaluation of atypical cases. This hernia may contain small bowel, colon, or omentum. The presence of bowel loops may be confirmed by visualization of valvulae conniventes, haustrations, and detection of peristalsis on real-time examinations. Hernias con-

taining omentum or other fatty masses will appear hyperechoic. If these features are absent, differentiation from other extratesticular masses such as hematocele and pyelocele would be difficult.[23, 29] (Courtesy of Kathy Toledo, Rhode Island Hospital, School of Diagnostic Medical Sonography, Providence, Rhode Island.)

74. C. Testicular torsion is due to a developmental weakness of the mesenteric attachment from the spermatic cord onto the testis and epididymis. It is common during adolescence but may occur at any age. Doppler ultrasound will show decreased arterial flow in the early hours following the incident. Eventually, the patient will demonstrate absence of intratesticular flow.[13]

75. B. The left epididymis appeared enlarged and hypoechoic. There was a small amount of fluid seen surrounding the testis on this side. The most common sonographic findings in epididymitis are of epididymal enlargement and decreased echogenicity. Other sonographic findings include scrotal skin thickening and a reactive hydrocele. Color Doppler will show increased blood flow due to tissue hyperemia. In epididymitis, the testicle is usually sonographically normal; however, if the inflammation is severe enough, testicular infarcts may be seen.[13]

REFERENCES

1. Arkfeld SJ, Rouse GA, DeLange M. Deep venous thrombosis of the lower extremity. J Diag Med Sonog 1991;7:2.

2. Bundy AL, Ritchie WGM. Inflammatory aneurysm of the abdominal aorta. J Clin Ultrasound 1984;12:102.

3. Buurma G. Guidelines for abdomen review. Dallas: Society of Diagnostic Medical Sonographers, 1990.

4. Ferguson GG. Pathophysiology: mechanisms and expressions. Philadelphia: WB Saunders, 1984.

5. Fornage BD, Sneige N, Faroux MJ, Andry E. Sonographic appearance and ultrasound-guided fine-needle aspiration biopsy of breast carcinomas smaller than 1 cm. J Ultrasound Med 1990;9:559.

6. Frazer HA. Ultrasound reduces miss rate for CDH in high-risk infants. Diagnostic Imaging 1989;Oct:37.

7. Goldenberg NJ, Spitz HB, Mitchell SE. Gray scale ultrasonography of the chest. Sem Ultrasound 1982;3(4):263.

8. Gooding GAW. Aneurysms of the abdominal aorta, iliac, and femoral arteries. Sem Ultrasound 1982;3(4):170.

9. Govan ADT, MacFarlane PS, Callander R. Pathology illustrated. Edinburgh: Churchill Livingstone, 1981.

10. Hall R. The ultrasound handbook. Philadelphia: JB Lippincott, 1988.

11. Hagen-Ansert SL. Textbook of diagnostic ultrasonography. St. Louis: CV Mosby, 1989.

12. Jeffrey RB. New imaging tools improve diagnosis of appendicitis. Diagnostic Imaging 1988;May:100.

13. Kawamura D. Diagnostic medical sonography. Vol 3: Abdomen. Philadelphia: JB Lippincott, 1992.

14. Mack LA, Matsen GA, Kilcoyne RF, et al. Ultrasound evaluation of the rotator cuff. Radiographics 1985;5:941.

15. McCann J. Researchers find novel applications for color Doppler. Diagnostic Imaging 1988;10:13.

16. McCarroll KA, Roszler MH. Drug abuse complications confront urban radiologists. Diagnostic Imaging 1989;Nov:268.

17. McGahan JP, ed. Controversies in ultrasound. In: Radiologic clinics of North America. Philadelphia: WB Saunders, 1985.

18. Miller EI, Rogers A. Sonography of the anterior abdominal wall. Sem Ultrasound 1982;3:278.

19. Netter FH. Ciba collection of medical illustrations. Vol 6. Rochester, New York: Case-Hoyt Corp, 1965.

20. Poljak A, Jeffrey RB, Kernberg ME. The gas-containing appendix: potential sonographic pitfalls in the diagnosis of acute appendicitis. J Ultrasound Med 1991;10:625.

21. Puylaert JBCM. Acute appendicitis: ultrasound evaluation using graded compression. Radiology 1986;158:355.

22. Robbin S. Basic pathology. Philadelphia: WB Saunders, 1987.

23. Rumack CM, Wilson SR, Charboneau JW. Diagnostic Ultrasound. Vol 1. St. Louis: Mosby Yearbook, 1991.

24. Sanders, RC. Clinical sonography: a practical guide. Boston: Little Brown, 1984.

25. Sarti DA. Diagnostic ultrasound: text and cases. Chicago: Year Book Medical Publishers, 1987.

26. Sauerbrei EE, Nguyen KT, Nolan RL. Abdominal sonography. New York: Raven Press, 1992.

27. Schroeder WB, Halec SW. The definitive assessment of aneurysm by color flow Doppler. J Diag Med Sonog 1991;7:201.

28. Slasky BS, Lenkey L, Skolnick ML, et al. Sonography of the soft tissues of extremities and trunk. Sem Ultrasound, 1982;3(4):288.

29. Teele R, Share JC. Ultrasonography of infants and children. Philadelphia: WB Saunders, 1991.

30. Tempkin BB. Ultrasound scanning: principles and protocols. Philadelphia: WB Saunders, 1993.

31. Westbrook CS, Rouse GA, DeLange M. Sonographic evaluation of the spine in infants and neonates. J Diag Med Sonog 1991;7:235.

Marveen Craig: *Ultrasound Exam Review*, © 1994 J. B. Lippincott Co.

4

Neonatal Neurosonography

OBJECTIVES

Neurosonography has undergone many important changes over the past 40 years. A-mode detection of midline shifts has given way to present day high-resolution, real-time, and Doppler examinations capable of producing precise intracranial detail and graphic evaluation of intracranial vascular performance. Use this chapter to test your knowledge of neuroanatomy, common pathologies, and special limitations associated with scanning the contents of the brain, and to reinforce your understanding of how to skillfully function within the confines of the neonatal intensive care facility.

QUESTIONS

Directions

Each of the questions or incomplete statements is followed by several answers or completions. Select the best answer(s) in each case. In the matching sections, answers should be used only once, unless otherwise stated.

1. The anterior fontanelle provides a valuable acoustic window for scanning the brain of the neonate. Closure of all fontanelles generally occurs by age:
   A. 6 months.
   B. 12 months.
   C. 18 months.
   D. 24 months.

2. Periventricular leukomalacia (PVL) initially presents a sonographic pattern of _____ echogenicity in the _____ area.
   A. increased; choroid plexus and ventricular atrium
   B. complex-cystic; occipital horns
   C. increased; frontal horns
   D. decreased; labyrinths

3. Because so much blood enters the head with a vein of Galen malformation, there is often associated:
   A. hydrops.
   B. heart failure.
   C. hydranencephaly.
   D. A and B

4. The V-shaped echogenic extension of the falx cerebri that separates the cerebrum and the cerebellum is known as the:
   A. tentorium.

B. trigone.
C. massa intermedia.
D. treponium.

5. Identify the numbered anatomical structures in Figure 4-1.

   1. ____   A. Thalamus
   2. ____   B. Occipital bone
   3. ____   C. Third ventricle
   4. ____   D. Caudate nucleus
   5. ____   E. Frontal horn

6. Dandy-Walker malformation describes a spectrum of disorders resulting from:
   A. an enlarged fourth ventricle and absent vermis.
   B. atresia of the foramina of Luschka and Magendie.
   C. fusion of the thalami.
   D. A and B

7. Factors increasing the risk of an

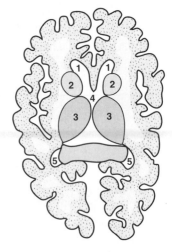

Figure 4-1. Neuroanatomy: axial section superior to the external auditory meatus.

intracranial bleed include all of the following *except:*
A. low birth weight.
B. ventriculitis.
C. traumatic delivery.
D. prematurity.

8. The sonolucent midline space lying inferior to the corpus callosum is the:
   A. fourth ventricle.
   B. cavum septum pellucidum.
   C. foramen of Monro.
   D. circle of Willis.

9. If an Arnold-Chiari malformation is suspected, the sonographic examination should also include the:
   A. brain stem.
   B. foramen magnum.
   C. spinal canal.
   D. vein of Galen.

10. Which of the following statements about neonatal neurosonography is *untrue?*
    A. Lateral ventricles will be demonstrated in the lower, medial portion of the cerebral hemispheres
    B. Each ventricle will contain a choroid plexus
    C. The caudate nucleus will appear less echogenic than the choroid plexi and the thalami
    D. Cerebral peduncles will appear at approximately the level of the external auditory meatus

11. Intracranial hemorrhage in premature infants develops in the:
    A. immature subependymal

germinal matrix of the caudate nucleus.
B. cerebellum and choroid plexus.
C. caudate nucleus.
D. all of the above

12. Permanent internal shunts are used to relieve the pressure of abnormal fluid collections within the ventricles. To ensure continued operation of the shunt it is important that the ventricular end be placed in the _____ portion of the lateral ventricle.
    A. anterior
    B. medial
    C. lateral
    D. posterior

13. Which of the following statements is *untrue* regarding neonatal sonography?
    A. Bilateral brain symmetry is best evaluated from coronal scan planes
    B. Duplex sonography is preferred
    C. Extensive patient preparation is required
    D. The scanhead should be supported with the fingers of one hand while the palm of that hand rests against the head

14. The grooves or depressions on the surface of the brain that separate its convolutions are called:
    A. sulci.
    B. gyri.
    C. vergi.
    D. clivi.

15. The most common complication associated with intracranial shunt function is the:
    A. embedment in the caudate nucleus.
    B. entanglement in the choroid plexus.
    C. damage of the shunt tubing.
    D. incorrect placement by the neurosurgeon.

16. Parenchymal hemorrhage eventually resolves and communicates with the lateral ventricle in the form of a
    A. choroid plexus cyst.
    B. subarachnoid cyst.
    C. myelin cyst.
    D. porencephalic cyst.

17. Identify the numbered anatomical structures in Figure 4-2.

    1. ___   A. Cerebral peduncle

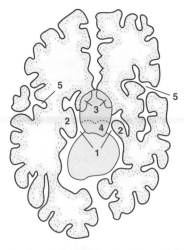

Figure 4-2. Neuroanatomy: axial section slightly superior to the external auditory meatus.

2. ___   B. Hippocampal gyrus
3. ___   C. Inferior colliculus
4. ___   D. Sylvian fissure
5. ___   E. Ambient cistern

18. Dilatation of the third and lateral ventricles only indicates obstruction:
    A. at the level of the arachnoid granulations.
    B. superior to the third ventricle.
    C. at the level of the foramen of Monro.
    D. at the level of the aqueduct of Sylvius.

19. Optimal sonographic detection and delineation of intracranial hemorrhage is best obtained with:
    A. frequencies of 5 MHz or greater.
    B. frequencies of 3.5 MHz.
    C. the highest frequency available.
    D. frequency of 25 MHz.

20. Which of the following are instrumentation artifacts encountered during neonatal neurosonography?
    A. Beam width or volume averaging
    B. Near-field reverberation, 60 cycle noise
    C. Attenuation
    D. All of the above

21. The subependymal growth plate is an area rich in blood vessels but poor in supporting structures in newborns. An-

other term used to describe this area is the:
A. cortical lobe.
B. caudate nuclei.
C. germinal matrix.
D. choroid plexi.

22. With a very small anterior fontanelle, it may not always be possible during parasagittal scanning to properly see the:
A. thalami.
B. occipital horns.
C. caudate nucleus.
D. third ventricle.

23. Subdural and primary subarachnoid hemorrhages usually occur in term infants as a result of:
A. anoxia.
B. infection.
C. birth trauma.
D. a defective clotting mechanism.

24. The optimal time for performing initial neurosonography of a preterm neonate is:
A. 1 week old.
B. 4–7 days old.
C. 2 weeks old.
D. as soon as possible after birth.

25. Select the correct definition of periventricular leukomalacia from the following choices.
A. Abscess formation within the white matter
B. Hardening of the white matter beside the lateral ventricle
C. Softening of the white matter beside the lateral ventricle

D. Accumulation of fluid following aneurysm rupture

26. Neonates undergoing neurosonography should be positioned:
A. with nose facing up.
B. with head down.
C. supine with head turned to right.
D. supine with head turned to left.

27. Which of the following structures would appear most echogenic?
A. Ventricles
B. Thalamus
C. Choroid plexus
D. Caudate nucleus

28. In a preterm neonate who shows sonographic evidence of mild periventricular hemorrhage, when should repeat sonographic studies be performed?
A. Every 3 days until age 2 weeks
B. Once weekly until age 2 weeks
C. Once weekly for 2 months
D. Every 3 days for 2 months

29. During sonographic imaging, the thalami are normally seen as:
A. single and square-shaped.
B. single and egg-shaped.
C. paired and square-shaped.
D. paired and egg-shaped.

30. Identify the numbered anatomical structures in Figure 4-3.

1. ___   A. Tentorium

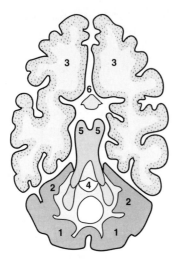

Figure 4-3. Neuroanatomy: axial section at the external auditory meatus level.

2. ___   B. Cerebral peduncle
3. ___   C. Cerebellum
4. ___   D. Circle of Willis
5. ___   E. Fourth ventricle
6. ___   F. Cerebrum

31. Some normal brain structures are capable of producing artifacts during neonatal neurosonography. They include the:
    A. thalami and cavum.
    B. falx and calcarine fissure.
    C. choroid plexus and caudate nucleus.
    D. vermis and major commisure.

32. Which of the following statements concerning arachnoid cysts is (are) *untrue?*
    A. Contain CSF
    B. Occur commonly near the sella
    C. Lie anterior to the third ventricle
    D. Contact the brain surface

33. Acute cerebral infarct follows a predictable course that can be followed with ultrasound. The most striking sonographic characteristics are hyperechogenicity and abnormal or loss of _____ definition.
    A. commissural
    B. sulci
    C. gyri
    D. B and C

34. In coronal views of agenesis of the corpus callosum, the ventricles will appear:
    A. elongated.
    B. parallel.
    C. shortened.
    D. perpendicular.

35. A Dandy-Walker cyst occurs in the subtentorial region of the brain and is characterized by absence of the cerebellar vermis. The Dandy-Walker cyst also communicates with the:
    A. fourth ventricle.
    B. germinal matrix.
    C. foramen of Monro.
    D. none of the above

36. Agenesis of the corpus callosum can result in partial or complete absence of the corpus callosum. Which of the following further characteristics is *not* associated with agenesis of the corpus callosum?
    A. Fusion of the thalami
    B. Abnormal pattern of sulci

on the interhemispheric surface
C. Fluid between the hemispheres
D. Lateral separation of the lateral ventricles, with beaking of the frontal horns

37. Intracranial calcifications are associated with:
   A. cytomegalo virus infection.
   B. tuberous sclerosis.
   C. toxoplasmosis.
   D. all of the above

38. Normal sulcal development occurs between _____ and _____ weeks:
   A. 28; 32
   B. 30; 38
   C. 32; 40
   D. 36; 40

39. Normal flow of the cerebral spinal fluid begins in the:
   A. cisterna magna.
   B. foramen of Magendie.
   C. foramen of Luschka.
   D. ventricles.

40. During sonographic examination of the posterior fossa, the transducer is placed on the anterior fontanelle in a coronal attitude. A good "starting" landmark would be pulsations of the circle of Willis, which is made up of the:
   A. basilar artery.
   B. communicating and cerebral arteries.
   C. internal carotid arteries.
   D. B and C

Match the following terms to numbers 41–58.
   A. Fontanelle
   B. Sulci
   C. Encephalomalacia
   D. Meninges
   E. Gyrus
   F. Quadrigeminal plate
   G. Arachnoid
   H. Ependyma
   I. Germinal matrix
   J. Aqueduct of Sylvius
   K. Massa intermedia
   L. Convolution
   M. Foramen of Monro
   N. Diencephalon
   O. Infarct
   P. Subarachnoid
   Q. Ischemia
   R. Choroid plexus

41. ____ A convolution of the cerebral cortex

42. ____ An echogenic structure immediately superior to the apex of the tentorium, resembling the top of a pine tree

43. ____ An elevated part of the surface of the brain

44. ____ A membranous spot in an infant's skull

45. ____ Portion of the brain lying between the cerebrum and midbrain

46. ____ Delicate web-like meninges

47. ____ Tissue necrosis caused by lack of blood supply

48. ___ Coverings of the brain and spinal cord

49. ___ Membrane lining ventricles and central spinal canal

50. ___ Area beneath the middle covering of brain and spinal cord

51. ___ Brain disease producing "softening" of the tissues

52. ___ Decreased blood supply

53. ___ Midline channel connecting third and fourth ventricles

54. ___ Midline channels that connect the third ventricle with each lateral ventricle

55. ___ Fissures of the brain

56. ___ Pea-shaped structure suspended within third ventricle

57. ___ Fragile periventricular tissue which includes the caudate nucleus

58. ___ Mass of specialized cells that regulate intra-ventricular pressure by secretion and absorption of cerebrospinal fluid

59. Identify the numbered anatomical structures in Figure 4-4.

1. ___   A. Midbrain
2. ___   B. Caudate nucleus

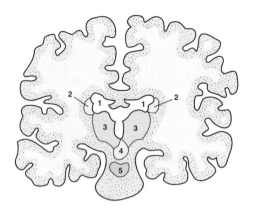

Figure 4-4. Neuroanatomy: coronal section of the midbrain.

3. ___   C. Ventricle
4. ___   D. Pons
5. ___   E. Trigone

60. The _____ lies anterior and superior to the thalamus.
    A. third ventricle
    B. hypothalamus
    C. peduncles
    D. caudate nucleus

61. Infants undergoing extracorporeal membrane oxygenation (ECMO) therapy are at risk for developing:
    A. hypoxic ischemic encephalopathy.
    B. cerebral edema, encephalomalacia.
    C. bilateral intraventricular hemorrhages.
    D. all of the above

62. The proper placement of the anterior tip of an intracranial shunt or reservoir is:
    A. in the frontal horn, posterior to the foramen of Monro.

B. in the frontal horn, anterior to the foramen of Monro.

C. in the body of the lateral ventricle, posterior to the foramen of Monro.

D. in the temporal horn, anterior to the foramen of Monro.

63. Select the primary uses of intraoperative neurosonography.
    A. Biopsy guidance and localization of intracerebral masses
    B. Localization of spinal cord masses
    C. Shunt placement
    D. A and B

64. The two internal cerebral veins unite posterior to the pineal gland to form the:
    A. superior cerebellar vein.
    B. meningeal vein.
    C. vein of Galen.
    D. inferior cerebellar vein.

65. Late stage central nervous system infections cause:
    A. ventriculitis and ventricular enlargement.
    B. intraventricular septations echogenic sulci.
    C. marked fontanelle expansion.
    D. A and B

66. The sonographic appearance of a large echo-free space surrounding the midbrain and absence of any cortical mantle is consistent with:
    A. hydranencephaly.
    B. holoprosencephaly.

C. encephalomalacia.
D. agenesis of the corpus callosum.

67. This coronal section of the brain (Fig. 4-5) demonstrates the thalamus (1) and third ventricle (2). Name the additional anatomical structure (3).
    A. Sylvian fissure
    B. Transverse fissure
    C. Calcerine fissure
    D. Longitudinal fissure

68. A proposed new position for scanning the infant cervical spine is:
    A. lateral decubitus, with knees flexed.
    B. prone, lying over the palm and forearm of the examiner.
    C. upright, flexed at the hips.
    D. lateral decubitus with legs extended.

69. Subependymal hemorrhage arises from the _____ , and bulges into the _____ .

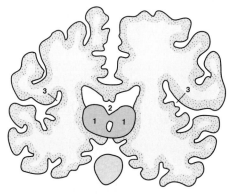

Figure 4-5. Neuroanatomy: coronal section of the midline structures.

A. central sulcus; parietal fissure
B. germinal matrix; lateral ventricle
C. diencephalon; pineal recess
D. corpus callosum; longitudinal fissure

70. The position of the conus medularis may be determined by counting up the vertebral bodies from the _____ lumbar vertebra.
    A. fourth
    B. fifth
    C. third
    D. second

71. What portion of the lateral ventricle is formed by the corpus callosum?
    A. Roof
    B. Medial
    C. Lateral
    D. Inferior

72. What anatomical structure connects the third and fourth ventricles?
    A. Aqueduct of Sylvius
    B. Foramen of Monro
    C. Foramen of Luschka
    D. Foramen of Magendie

73. What anatomical structure connects the third ventricle to the lateral ventricles?
    A. Aqueduct of Sylvius
    B. Foramen of Monro
    C. Foramen of Luschka
    D. Foramen of Magendie

74. Sonographic intracranial findings associated with the Dandy-Walker malformation may include all of the following *except:*
    A. hypoplastic cerebellar vermis.
    B. elevation of the tentorium.
    C. hydrocephalus.
    D. enlargement of the massa intermedia.

75. Neonatal sonographers may encounter normal variants during scanning. Most normal variants are due to gestational immaturity. Which of the following is (are) commonly recognized normal intracranial variants?
    A. Lateral ventricular disparity
    B. Periventricular "halos"
    C. Asymmetry of the occipital horns
    D. All of the above

76. Dandy-Walker malformation is thought to be the result of:
    A. neural tube defects.
    B. malformation of the roof of the fourth ventricle.
    C. arachnoid septations.
    D. cerebrospinal fluid stasis.

77. Fetal anomalies associated with Dandy-Walker malformation include all of the following *except:*
    A. agenesis of the corpus callosum.
    B. aqueductal stenosis.
    C. encephalocele.
    D. holoprosencephaly.

78. Which type of holoprosencephaly has the worst prognosis?

A. Alobar
B. Semilobar
C. Lobar
D. Quadri lobar

79. The sonographic features of alobar holoprosencephaly include all of the following *except:*
   A. agenesis of the corpus callosum.
   B. an intact falx cerebri.
   C. a fused thalami.
   D. a proboscis.

80. Holoprosencephaly carries a high risk of underlying chromosomal abnormalities. The most common chromosomal abnormality associated with holoprosencephaly is:
   A. trisomy 13.
   B. trisomy 21.
   C. trisomy 18.
   D. Down's syndrome.

CASES AND QUESTIONS

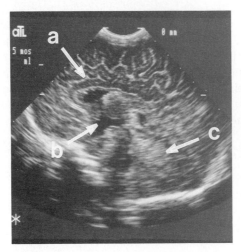

Figure 4-6. Midline sagittal sonogram of the neonatal cranium. (Courtesy of Michelle Guillory, Ochsner Medical Foundation, New Orleans, Louisiana.)

Scans of a normal 5-month-old infant.

81. Identify the structure indicated by the arrow *a* in Figure 4-6.
    A. Thalamus
    B. Third ventricle
    C. Lateral ventricle
    D. Corpus callosum

82. Identify arrow *b* on Figure 4-6.
    A. Thalamus
    B. Third ventricle
    C. Fourth ventricle
    D. Lateral ventricle

83. Arrow *c* in Figure 4-6 represents the:
    A. cerebellum.
    B. fourth ventricle.
    C. peduncles.
    D. cisterna magna.

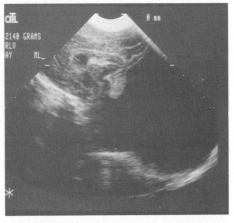

A

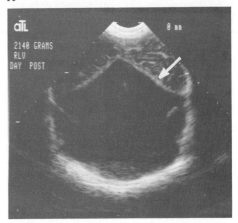

B

Figure 4-7. (*A*) Sagittal sonogram of the neonatal brain. (*B*) Coronal sonogram of the neonatal brain. (Courtesy of Benita Barthel, Ochsner Medical Foundation, New Orleans, Louisiana.)

The patient, a 1-day-old infant, was delivered at 34 weeks' gestation because of increasing hydrocephalus. Obstetrical sonography had demonstrated the presence of a posterior fossa cyst. Cranial ultrasound was performed at about 1 day of age, and revealed a large posterior fossa cyst. Neither the cerebellum nor the fourth ventricle was well seen. The third and lateral ventricles were noted to be dilated. The corpus callosum was hard to identify.

84. The diagnosis that can be made from information contained in Figure 4-7A is that of a (an):
    A. enlarged cisterna magna.
    B. arachnoid cyst.
    C. Chiari II malformation.
    D. Dandy-Walker cyst.

85. The arrow indicated on Figure 4-7B points to the:
    A. fourth ventricle.
    B. hippocampal gyri.
    C. tentorium.
    D. falx cerebri.

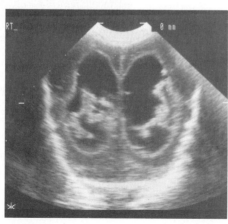

A

Figure 4-8. (A) Coronal and (B) Sagittal brain scans of a premature infant taken 25 days after birth. (Courtesy of Richard Lane, Palm Beach Community College, Palm Beach Gardens, Florida.)

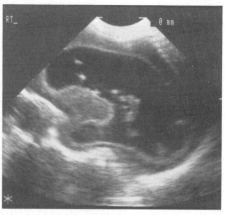

B

Figure 4-8. (continued)

This patient was a premature infant (24-weeks' gestation; Apgar score of 5:7) weighing 1 lb 3 oz, with hyaline membrane disease. Approximately 1 week after birth the infant became unstable and received several transfusions for anemia. At 2 weeks of age the infant demonstrated increased stiffness and muscle tone in the legs.

86. The scans in Figure 4-8 demonstrate sonographic evidence of:
    A. subependymal cysts.
    B. porencephalic cysts.
    C. subgerminal, interventricular hemorrhage.
    D. edematous brain.

87. The intracranial sonographic findings demonstrated in Figure 4-9 are consistent with:
    A. hydranencephaly.
    B. holoprosencephaly.
    C. megalencephaly.
    D. schizencephaly.

88. Epidural hematomas typically occur in the term infant. The

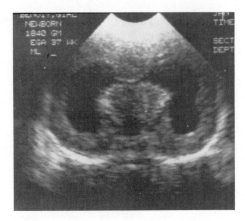

Figure 4-9. Coronal sonogram of the neonatal brain. (Courtesy of Benita Barthel, Ochsner Medical Foundation, New Orleans, Louisiana.)

cause of epidural hematoma is rupture of a meningeal artery, which leads to an accumulation of arterial blood between the _____ and the _____ .

   A. dura; brain

   B. dura; skull

   C. brain; superior sagittal sinus

   D. A or C

89. A Grade III intracranial hemorrhage is one that:

   A. is confined to the germinal matrix.

   B. causes extravasation of blood into the ventricles.

   C. produces dilated, blood-filled ventricles.

   D. is associated with concurrent intraparenchymal bleeding.

90. To minimize the dangers of thermal stress when performing neonatal neurosonography,

which of the following procedures should be observed?

   A. Contact media (scanning gel) should be warmed

   B. Scanning gel should immediately be removed upon completion of scan

   C. Close the portholes at the end of the procedure

   D. All of the above

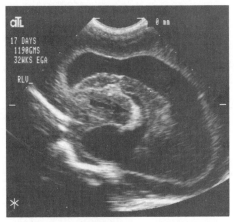

Figure 4-10. Sagittal sonogram of the right lateral ventricle. (Courtesy of Dixie Alexander, Ochsner Medical Foundation, New Orleans, Louisiana.)

Sonographic study of an 1190-gram neonate born at 32 weeks' gestation. No other cranial studies were performed.

91. Based on the information contained in Figure 4-10, select the appropriate diagnosis.

   A. Intracranial hemorrhage, Grade I

   B. Intracranial hemorrhage, Grade II

C. Intracranial hemorrhage, Grade III
D. Intracranial hemorrhage, Grade IV

92. Factors associated with an increased risk for intracranial bleeding include all of the following *except:*
    A. low birth weight.
    B. ventriculitis.
    C. traumatic delivery.
    D. prematurity.

93. The most common timing for intracranial bleeding in premature infants occurs:
    A. during birth.
    B. 24 hours after birth.
    C. 36 hours after birth.
    D. 72 hours after birth.

Sonographic brain scans were ordered on a premature infant who, at 74 days old, weighed 2000 grams. No other cranial studies were performed.

94. Identify the structure in Figure 4-11 labeled (1).
    A. Choroid plexus
    B. Corpus callosum
    C. Cerebellum
    D. Thalamus

95. Identify structure (2) in Figure 4-11.
    A. Choroid plexus
    B. Corpus callosum
    C. Cerebellum
    D. Thalamus

96. What anatomical structure lies between (1) and (2)?
    A. Third ventricle
    B. Lateral ventricle
    C. Foramen of Monro
    D. Hypothalamus

97. The findings in Figure 4-11 are consistent with:
    A. evidence of a subarachnoid hemorrhage.
    B. evidence of a subependymal hemorrhage.
    C. evidence of a choroid plexus hemorrhage.
    D. no evidence of hemorrhage.

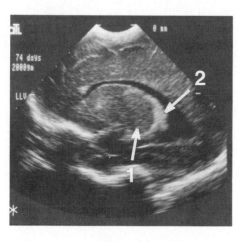

Figure 4-11. Sagittal scan of the left ventricle. (Courtesy of Michelle Guillory, Ochsner Medical Foundation, New Orleans, Louisiana.)

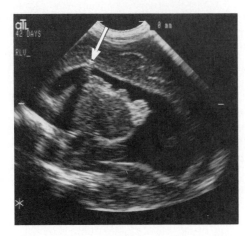

Figure 4-12. Sagittal scan of the left lateral ventricle. (Courtesy of Alicia Fernandez, Ochsner Medical Foundation, New Orleans, Louisiana.)

Neurosonographic study of a 1190-gram neonate, born at 32 weeks' gestation, currently being treated for posthemorrhagic hydrocephalus.

98. The arrow in Figure 4-12 points to:

A. residual clot.
B. intracranial shunt or reservoir.
C. normal cerebrospinal fluid.
D. brain sulci.

99. The most common causes of intraventricular hydrocephalus include all of the following *except:*
A. aqueductal stenosis.
B. intracranial hemorrhage.
C. choroid plexus papilloma.
D. Dandy-Walker malformation.

100. When only the third and lateral ventricles display signs of dilation, obstruction is most likely to be found:
A. superior to the third ventricle.
B. at the level of the circle of Willis.
C. at the level of the Retzian space.
D. at the level of the Sylvian aqueduct.

ANSWERS

1. C. Fontanelles are spaces between the bones of the skulls of neonates and infants. The anterior fontanelle in the baby lies between the two halves of the frontal bone in front and the two parietal bones behind. It is usually no longer palpable after 18 months.[17]

2. C. Periventricular leukomalacia results from an ischemic insult (often sustained during labor) and results in the diffuse cerebral infarction and necrosis of brain tissue. Initially PVL produces a hyperechoic appearance in the region of the frontal horns. This increased echogenic pattern can extend into the cerebrum. The damaged area eventually becomes less echogenic with the process of cystic liquefaction (approximately 1–3 weeks later).[8]

3. D. An infant in cardiac failure without detectable heart lesions suggests the possibility of a large-volume arteriovenous shunt. Such malformations are frequently associated with heart failure and cyanosis. Of these, many will involve the vein of Galen. Evidence of high output failure such as cardiomegaly, enlarged neck veins, or hydrops predicts a poor outcome. The sonographic appearance of a vein of Galen arteriovenous malformation typically is of a well-defined circular, oval, or cigar-shaped sonolucency in the quadrigeminal cistern. Often, the location and number of abnormal vessels render the malformation inoperable and death follows from intractable heart failure.[4,14,18]

4. A. The outermost meningeal covering of the brain is the dura mater, which has two layers. In most places, these layers are in contact with each other, but in other areas the internal dura sends extensions into some of the fissures of the brain while the external dura remains close to the interior of the skull. The falx cerebri, a fold of dura (in the longitudinal fissure), forms the superior sagittal sinus. The *tentorium cerebelli* (which lies in the transverse fissure) forms the straight sinuses in its folds. These sinuses contain venous blood that will ultimately flow into the internal jugular veins.[2]

5. 1. E, 2. D, 3. A, 4. C, 5. B[15,17]

6. C. A Dandy-Walker malformation consists of congenital cystic dilation of the fourth ventricle due to atresia of the foramina of Luschka and Magendie, along with hypoplastic cerebellar hemispheres and hypoplastic or absent vermis.[16,18] (Courtesy of Laura Arteaga, Orange Coast College, Costa Mesa, California.)

7. B. Clinical symptoms that make a pediatrician suspicious of intracranial hemorrhage include prematurity, respiratory distress syndrome (RDS), a drop in hematocrit, a low birth weight (under 1500 g), and trauma at delivery.[16] (Courtesy of Dixie Alexander, Ochsner Medical Foundation, New Orleans, Louisiana.)

8. B. The cavum septum pellucidum (anterior portion) is a midline, anechoic, fluid-filled structure projecting superoanterior to the third ventricle and lying inferior to the corpus callosum.[19]

9. C. Arnold-Chiari malformation is associated with spina bifida and myelomeningocele. In a neonate the spinal canal should be examined to make sure that no intraspinal mass is present and the cord does not extend too low.[16,18]

10. C. The caudate nucleus is located within the concavity of the lateral angles of each lateral ventricle and produces medium-level echoes.[16,19]

11. D. The majority of preterm neonatal intracranial hemorrhages occur in the periventricular-intraventricular areas of the brain (the germinal matrix, caudate nucleus, cerebellum, choroid plexus).[1,14,16] (Courtesy of Carrie Lundy, Orange Coast College, Costa Mesa, California.)

12. A. The ventricular end of a shunt is usually placed in the anterior horn of the lateral ventricle, anterior to the foramen of Monro. Such placement will ensure that the choroid plexus cannot block the tip or side holes of the shunt, since the choroid plexus is located in the ventricular atrium.[14]

13. C. Patient preparation for neonatal brain scanning requires several simple safeguards: keeping the infant warm and the coupling gel at body temperature; disturbing the infant as little as possible—preferably leaving him or her in the isolette; safeguarding the infant by wearing gowns and gloves and cleaning the portable ultrasound system with an appropriate cleansing agent.[19]

14. A. The sulci are echogenic, spider-like fissures separating the gyri or folds of the brain. They appear fewer in number in the premature neonate.[19]

15. B. One of the common complications of a shunt is its capacity to become entangled in the choroid plexus when it slips out of position.[13,14] (Courtesy of Alicia Fernandez, Ochsner Medical Foundation, New Orleans, Louisiana.)

16. D. Intraparenchymal hemorrhage usually resolves leaving behind a porencephalic cyst.[16]

17. 1. E, 2. B, 3. A, 4. C, 5. D[15,17]

18. D. When obstruction of cerebral-spinal fluid (CSF) is confined to the lateral ventricles, obstruction at the level of the aqueduct of Sylvius is indicated.[13,14] (Courtesy of Alicia Fernandez, Ochsner Medical Foundation, New Orleans, Louisiana.)

19. A. For optimum results a high-frequency (5 MHz or more), high-resolution, real-time scanner is preferred. The transducer should be placed on the anterior fontanelle and "rotated" to provide both coronal and sagittal scan planes.[19]

20. D. Beamwidth or volume averaging artifacts occur because ultrasound instruments are designed to assume that all returning echoes originate from the central axis of the sound beam. In reality, the beam returns echoes of varying intensities arising from interfaces at many locations. When all returning echoes within the sound beam are averaged and placed along the central axis, the actual anatomy may be misrepresented. Near-field artifacts can be avoided by using water path techniques so that the brain or spinal cord tissue can be adequately visualized in the optimum zone of the near field. Attenuation of the beam by bone presents a problem. Since ultrasound systems are calibrated for the speed of sound in tissue (1540 m/s) and the velocity of sound in bone (4080 m/s) is faster, it is possible that returning echoes will be incorrectly placed on the image as registration errors. Improper grounding of an ultrasound unit can result in sensitive receivers picking up line noise of 60 cycles per second from other nearby equipment in the intensive care unit. Noise degrades the image, appearing within it as echo-streaks or linear dots.[6,10]

21. C. The germinal matrix is situated along the inferior aspect of the lateral ventricles, immediately beneath the ependymal lining of the ventricle, and extends from the frontal horn backwards, into the occipital horn area.[11,17]

22. B. Performing parasagittal scans through a small anterior fontanelle may make it difficult to adequately image the region of the occipital horn. This area is critically important because it is where blood frequently collects.[16]

23. C. Subdural and primary subarachnoid hemorrhages usually occur in term infants following birth trauma.[14]

24. B. In preterm neonates, an initial real-time sonographic study should be done between the ages of 4 and 7 days.[1]

25. C. Periventricular leukomalacia can be defined as the softening of the white matter beside the lateral ventricle. Usually occurring in premature neonates who have suffered from asphyxia, this softening is due to ischemic infarction of the brain tissues. Hemorrhage may or may not occur into this ischemic tissue.[8,18]

26. A. For sonographic examination of the neonatal brain the infant should be positioned on its back with the nose facing upward to allow maximum contact of the transducer with the anterior fontanelle.[7,16,19]

27. C. The choroid plexus appears as a highly echogenic structure lying within the ventricle.[14,16]

28. A. In a preterm infant in whom hemorrhage has been demonstrated, sonographic studies should be repeated every 3 days until the age of 2 weeks, in order to follow the progression of the hemorrhage.[1,14]

29. D. The thalami usually appear as oval-, delta-wing-, or egg-shaped structures on either side of the third ventricle.[16] (Courtesy of Michelle Guillory, Ochsner Medical Foundation, New Orleans, Louisiana.)

30. 1. C, 2. A, 3. F, 4. E, 5. B, 6. D[15,17]

31. B. Normal intracerebral structures occasionally generate artifacts. The falx cerebri lies directly inferior to the anterior fontanelle, and therefore, directly beneath the central axis of the sound beam when the transducer is positioned in the midline. Occasionally, the falx will generate a shadow that overlies the third ventricle. Demonstration of the third ventricle can then be achieved by rocking the transducer slightly to one side of the midline and then angling back to it. During sagittal scanning of the occipital horns, an echogenicity is occasionally demonstrated within them and appears to be continuous with the choroid plexus. These occipital horn echoes may be a clot or echoes from the calcarine fissure projected into the occipital horn. Careful correction of the parasagittal scan plane (laterally) should enable visualization of the occipital horns free of any artifact. Echoes generated from a true clot will appear on coronal as well as sagittal scans.[10]

32. C. Arachnoid cysts, containing cerebral spinal fluid (CSF), result from adhesions of the meninges. Fluid is usually trapped in the cistern areas (particularly of the sella turcica) *posterior* to the third ventricle and posterior fossa.[8]

33. D. Acute cerebral infarct is characterized by hyperechogenicity and abnormal sulci and gyri. Vascular pulsations also disappear, but may return in the more chronic stages when the brain becomes revascularized. At that same time hypoechoic areas can be seen, which correspond pathologically to cysts.[3, 14, 18]

34. B. Agenesis of the corpus callosum can be noted as paralleling ventricles on coronal views, often with an associated high-riding third ventricle. The pathognomonic sagittal image is that of an absent corpus callosum and gyri that run perpendicular, rather than parallel, to the ventricles.[3]

35. A. A Dandy-Walker cyst produces dilation of the fourth ventricle as a result of atresia of the foramina of Luschka and Magendie. A posterior fossa cyst may extend out into the occipital region. The fourth-ventricle cyst occupies the area where the cerebellum usually lies, with secondary dilatation occurring in the third and lateral ventricles.[16]

36. A. The corpus callosum normally forms the roof of the lateral ventricles. Agenesis occurs when bundles of callosal fibers (Probst's bundles) parallel each other and do not connect across the midline.[3, 14, 16]

37. D. In general, infections such as cytomegalic inclusion disease and toxoplasmosis, and diseases such as tuberous sclerosis and dystrophic changes secondary to anoxia (infarct), will lead to intracranial calcifications.[18]

38. C. Normal sulcal development occurs between 32 and 40 weeks. Among the first to be formed are the parieto-occipital sulcus, which carries the middle cerebral artery, and the cingulate sulcus, which carries the callosal marginal artery. Many more sulci and vessels develop as the infant matures. Absence of sulci in term infants suggests the presence of cerebral edema or infection.[14]

39. D. Cerebrospinal fluid is produced by the choroid plexuses within the lateral, third, and fourth ventricles of the brain. It escapes from the ventricular system of the brain through the three foramina in the roof of the fourth ventricle and so enters the subarachnoid space.[10, 17]

40. D. The circle of Willis is formed by nine arteries: the anterior communicating artery, both anterior cerebral arteries, both internal carotid arteries, both posterior communicating arteries, and both posterior cerebral arteries. The circle of Willis allows blood that enters by either internal carotid or vertebral arteries to be distributed to any part of both cerebral hemispheres. Cortical and central branches arise from the circle and supply the brain substance.[1, 2, 14, 15, 17]

41. E

42. I

43. L

44. A

45. N

46. G

47. O

48. D

49. H

50. P

51. C

52. Q

53. J

54. M

55. B

56. K

57. R

58. F[11, 16, 17, 19]

59. 1. C, 2. B, 3. E, 4. A, 5. D[15, 17]

60. D. The caudate nucleus, which forms the lateral borders of the frontal horn of the lateral ventricle, lies anterior to the thalamus.[16] (Courtesy of Michelle Guillory, Ochsner Medical Foundation, New Orleans, Louisiana.)

61. D. Serial neurosonography can help alert physicians to hypoxic ischemia and other complications (cerebral edema, encephalomalacia, and intraventricular hemorrhage) resulting from extracorporeal membrane oxygenation (ECMO) in infants.[18]

62. B. The anterior tip of a shunt or reservoir should be placed in the frontal horn, anterior to the foramen of Monro.[10, 16] (Courtesy of Alicia Fernandez, Ochsner Medical Foundation, New Orleans, Louisiana.)

63. D. Intraoperative neurosonography has proven valuable in localizing brain or spinal cord masses and sonographically guiding a biopsy needle.[12]

64. C. The two internal cerebral veins unite just posterior to the pineal gland to form the great vein of Galen, which then courses posteriorly to empty into the straight sinus.[4]

65. D. Inflammation of the ventricles extends to the choroid plexus and ependymal lining. The choroid becomes misshapened and the walls of the ventricle appear thickened. Septations develop, dividing the ventricles into separate compartments. Moderate to extensive ventricular enlargement can occur. The sulcal echoes may also widen and increase in brightness.[14]

66. A. In hydranencephaly the cortical brain structures are absent. Only the midbrain and brainstem tissues are present, surrounded by fluid.[16]

67. A. The surface layer of each hemisphere is called the cortex and is composed of gray matter. The cerebral cortex is thrown into folds, or gyri, separated by fissures, or sulci. A number of the large sulci are conveniently used to subdivide the surface of each hemisphere into lobes. The Sylvian, or lateral, fissure is a deep fissure that separates the parietal and frontal lobes from the temporal lobe.[17]

68. B. The simple maneuver of holding the infant prone across the arm and flexing the neck allows good visualization of the cervical spine. There are several advantages to scanning the cervical spine using this technique: first, flexing the cervical spine splays the posterior elements, widening the intersegmental spaces for better sound transmission. Second, the spine is straightened, allowing use of a high-frequency linear-array transducer rather than a narrow-sector angle-scanning head. It is important that before flexing the neck of a newborn infant with suspected craniocervical anomalies, the cervical spine be evaluated with plain films so that spinal cord or nerve injury can be avoided. Also, care must be taken not to flex the neck excessively or compromise the infant's airway.[9]

69. B. Subependymal hemorrhage arises from the germinal matrix and bulges into the lateral ventricle. It does not rupture the overlying ependyma of the ventricle, hence the term *subependymal*.[14, 16, 17]

70. B. A tethered spinal cord produces abnormally low placement of the conus medularis tip, which lies below the level of the third lumbar vertebral body. Sonography can demonstrate the low position of the conus by counting up the vertebral bodies from the fifth lumbar vertebra.[20]

71. A. The roof of the anterior horn of the lateral ventricle is formed by

the body of the corpus callosum.[14, 17] (Courtesy of Michelle Guillory, Ochsner Medical Foundation, New Orleans, Louisiana.)

72. A. The cerebral aqueduct is a narrow channel, approximately 1 cm long, that connects the third and fourth ventricles. It is also known as the aqueduct of Sylvius.[14] (Courtesy of Michelle Guillory, Ochsner Medical Foundation, New Orleans, Louisiana.)

73. B. The foramen of Monro, which is also known as the interventricular foramen, provides communication between the lateral and third ventricles.[14] (Courtesy of Michelle Guillory, Ochsner Medical Foundation, New Orleans, Louisiana.)

74. D. The massa intermedia, located within the third ventricle, is not related to Dandy-Walker abnormalities.[14] (Courtesy of Benita Barthel, Ochsner Medical Foundation, New Orleans, Louisiana.)

75. D. Frequently, one lateral ventricle will appear larger than the other. If the disparity is too great, pathology should be suspected, and serial studies should be performed on borderline cases. Most neonates demonstrate asymmetry of the occipital horns. Normal variants include bilateral or unilateral absence, and differences in size when both are present. The entire ventricular system appears larger in the preterm neonate; in the very immature neonate the anterior horns are larger than in the term neonate. The "halo" seen around the lateral ventricles is most pronounced in the region of the trigone and is visible on most neonatal scans. A normal halo is never as echogenic as the glomus of the choroid plexus; whereas, pathologic conditions such as periventricular leukomalacia are as "bright" as the choroid glomus.[10, 14]

76. B. Atresia of the foramina of the fourth ventricle is usually called the Dandy-Walker deformity.[11, 14] (Courtesy of Benita Barthel, Ochsner Medical Foundation, New Orleans, Louisiana.)

77. D. Holoprosencephaly results from failure of cleavage of the prosencephalon.[3, 10] (Courtesy of Benita Barthel, Ochsner Medical Foundation, New Orleans, Louisiana.)

78. A. Infants with alobar holoprosencephaly generally have numerous associated defects or anomalies (facial deformities, encephaloceles, cystic hygroma, limb defects, etc.). Death usually occurs during the first year.[14, 17] (Courtesy of Benita Barthel, Ochsner Medical Foundation, New Orleans, Louisiana.)

79. B. With alobar holoprosencephaly, the telencephalon remains as a single cerebral hemisphere with one central ventricle. No falx, longitudinal fissure, or corpus callosum develop. The diencephalon fails to separate into two thalami. However, the cerebellum and brainstem may be normal.[10, 14, 16] (Courtesy of Benita Barthel, Ochsner Medical Foundation, New Orleans, Louisiana.)

80. A. In virtually any CNS anomaly, an analysis of the karyotype should be considered. A karyotype is clearly indicated in the case of holoprosencephalies, where a high incidence of chromosomal abnormalities have been discovered. Trisomy 13 is particularly common.[5, 13] (Courtesy of Benita Barthel, Ochsner Medical Foundation, New Orleans, Louisiana.)

81. D. The corpus callosum lies in the longitudinal fissure. It is a fibrous structure that connects the cerebral hemispheres.[14]

82. B. The narrow, slit-like, echo-free structure is the third ventricle.

83. B. The fourth ventricle is an irregularly shaped cavity located in the rhombencephalon.[14, 17]

84. D. The sonographic diagnosis was of a Dandy-Walker cyst. A CT scan of the head was performed 1 week later and demonstrated a large posterior fossa CSF density that communicated with the fourth ventricle and was thought to represent a Dandy-Walker malformation. Associated cerebellar hypoplasia and elevated tentorium secondary to hydrocephalus was also demonstrated. The cavum septum pellucidum was seen, and no discrete evidence of collosal agenesis was noted. The infant received a shunt and had multiple shunt revision for malfunction. The infant died at age 8 months.

85. C

86. C. These scans were taken from one of numerous serial studies performed on the infant from day 1 through day 35. Day 1 studies revealed normal intracranial findings but by days 3 to 7 echoes were seen within the ventricles (bilaterally), consistent with intraventricular hemorrhage. Figure 4-9 represents a study performed at day 25, one week following a lumbar spinal tap. It demonstrates continued and increasing presence of fluid and hemorrhagic material within the ventricles, consistent with subgerminal, intraventricular hemorrhage.

87. B. Holoprosencephaly results from failure of the prosencephalon to

diverticulate and produces a sonographic pattern of a U-shaped, single ventricle overlying fused or partially fused thalamic structures, and only thin cortical mantle echoes.[14, 17]

88. B. Epidural hematoma leads to the accumulation of arterial blood between the dura and the skull. Subdural hematoma results from damage to the veins between the brain and the superior sagittal sinus, and leads to the accumulation of blood between the dura and the brain.[10, 14] (Courtesy of Benita Barthel, Ochsner Medical Foundation, New Orleans, Louisiana.)

89. C. Most grading systems for evaluation of intracranial hemorrhage are modifications of the work of Burstein and Papile in 1978. A Grade I hemorrhage is isolated to the region of the germinal matrix; Grade II describes subependymal (SEH) or choroid plexus (CPH) and intraventricular hemorrhage (IVH)—but without ventricular dilatation; Grade III represents SEH or CPH with the addition of ventricular dilatation; Grade IV consists of SEH or CPH with IVH and intraparenchymal hemorrhage.[14] (Courtesy of Benita Barthel, Ochsner Medical Foundation, New Orleans, Louisiana.)

90. D. Because a newborn's head represents 2% of its total body surface area and is a significant source of heat loss, it is important to use warm gel during cranial sonography, remove the gel as soon as the scans are completed, and close the portholes of the isolette immediately upon completion of the ultrasound study to diminish the amount of heat loss.[10]

91. C.[14, 16]

92. B. Ventriculitis, an inflammatory rather than a traumatic condition, is not commonly associated with hemorrhagic consequences.[16] (Courtesy of Dixie Alexander, Ochsner Medical Foundation, New Orleans, Louisiana.)

93. D. Most incidences of intracranial bleeding in premature infants occurs at approximately 72 hours following birth.[16] (Courtesy of Dixie Alexander, Ochsner Medical Foundation, New Orleans, Louisiana.)

94. D.

95. A.

96. A.[14]

97. D. No evidence of hemorrhage is present in this image.

98. B.

99. C. A choroid plexus papilloma is an uncommon neoplastic growth that is not associated with intracranial bleeding.[14] (Courtesy of Alicia Fernandez, Ochsner Medical Foundation, New Orleans, Louisiana.)

100. D.[14] (Courtesy of Alicia Fernandez, Ochsner Medical Foundation, New Orleans, Louisiana.)

REFERENCES

1. Babcock DS. Cranial ultrasound of infants. Baltimore: Williams & Wilkins, 1981.

2. Burke SR. Anatomy and physiology for the health sciences. New York: John Wiley & Sons, 1980.

3. Cohen HL, Ziprkowski MN. New diagnostic insights in pediatric neurosonography. Diagnostic Imaging, November 1991;142.

4. Comstock CH, Kirk JS. Arteriovenous malformations. J Ultrasound Med 1991; 10:361.

5. Callen P. Ultrasonography in obstetrics and gynecology. Philadelphia: WB Saunders, 1983.

6. Edelman S. Understanding ultrasound physics. Houston: ESP Publishers, 1990.

7. Hagen-Ansert SL. Textbook of diagnostic ultrasonography. 3rd ed. St. Louis: CV Mosby, 1989.

8. Hall R. The ultrasound handbook. Philadelphia: JB Lippincott, 1988.

9. Harlow CL, Drose JA. A special technique for cervical spine sonography. J Ultrasound Med 1992;11:502.

10. McCann M. Neurosonology. Winnipeg, Canada: Burwin DMS Services, 1992.

11. Moore KL. The developing human. 2nd ed. Philadelphia: WB Saunders, 1977.

12. Pleitez GA, Rouse GA, DeLange M. Intraoperative spinal sonography. J Diag Med Sonog 1992;8:310.

13. Rumack CM, Wilson ST, Charboneau WJ. Diagnostic ultrasound. St. Louis: Mosby Year Book, 1991.

14. Rumack CM, Johnson M. Perinatal and infant brain imaging. Chicago: Year Book Medical Publishers, 1984.

15. Rumack CM, Horgan JG, Hay TC, Kindsfater D. Pocket atlas of pediatric ultrasound. New York: Raven Press, 1990.

16. Sanders RC. Clinical sonography: a practical guide. 2nd ed. Boston: Little Brown, 1991.

17. Snell RS. Clinical anatomy for medical students. Boston: Little Brown, 1973.

18. Teele R, Share JC. Ultrasonography of infants and children. Philadelphia: WB Saunders, 1991.

19. Tempkin BB. Ultrasound scanning: principles and protocols. Philadelphia: WB Saunders, 1993.

20. Westbrook CS, Rouse GA, DeLange M. Sonographic evaluation of the spine in infants and neonates. J Diag Med Sonog 1991;7:325.

5

Obstetrics and Gynecology

OBJECTIVES

The past decade has produced impressive technological advances in obstetric and gynecologic sonography. Tied to that advancement, however, is the sonographer's commitment to keep pace through continuous expansion of technical and clinical knowledge. This chapter is designed to focus on the changing depth and breadth of knowledge required of today's sonographers. It is intended not simply to aid them in achieving successful test scores but to help them meet the increasingly challenging demands placed upon them.

QUESTIONS

Directions

Each of the questions or incomplete statements is followed by several answers or completions. Select the best answer(s) in each case. In the matching sections, answers should be used only once, unless otherwise stated.

1. Intrauterine life is subdivided into the period of the ovum, the period of the embryo, and the period of the fetus. The embryonic period occurs from weeks _____ through _____ .
   A. 2; 6
   B. 3; 8
   C. 5; 9
   D. 6; 12

2. Ovarian size is related to a patient's age and phase of follicular development. The ovaries of postmenopausal women are usually smaller than those of premenopausal women because of:
   A. diminished circulation.
   B. diminished estrogen.
   C. diminished follicle stimulating hormone (FSH).
   D. A and B

3. The macrosomic fetus of a diabetic woman can be differentiated from that of a nondiabetic woman by measuring:
   A. biparietal diameter (BPD) and femur length (FL).
   B. liver size and fetal weight.
   C. thigh circumference.
   D. nuchal thickening.

4. The umbilical arteries arise from the fetal:
   A. abdominal aorta.
   B. portal vein.
   C. external iliac arteries.
   D. internal iliac arteries.

5. The most common site for fertilization is within the:
   A. distal third of the tube.
   B. proximal third of the tube.
   C. cornua of the uterus.
   D. fundus of the uterus.

6. Name the substance that surrounds and protects the vessels within the umbilical cord.
   A. Cerebral spinal fluid
   B. Amniotic fluid
   C. Wharton's jelly
   D. Petroleum jelly

7. The existence of only a single ventricle and fused thalami manifest the most severe form of:
   A. Kleebattschädel syndrome.
   B. hydranencephaly.
   C. Arnold-Chiari syndrome.
   D. holoprosencephaly.

8. Normal human cells contain _____ pairs of chromosomes.
   A. 21
   B. 23
   C. 24
   D. 26

9. The patient is a 22-year-old female with a history of a blocked fallopian tube. Sonography dem-

onstrates a mass in the cul-de-sac accompanied by free-fluid. The sonographer should:
A. check the hCG levels for this patient.
B. look for signs of intrauterine pregnancy.
C. examine the ovaries for possible endometriosis.
D. A and B

10. In a middle-aged female with a prior history of colon cancer and a current finding of pelvoabdominal mass, the sonographer should look for signs of:
A. Sertoli-Leydig tumor.
B. Krukenberg tumors.
C. cystadenocarcinoma of the ovaries.
D. endometrial involvement of the ovaries.

11. A corpus luteum cyst can be differentiated from a follicle cyst by observing a:
A. smooth, internal cyst wall pattern.
B. crenelated inner wall pattern.
C. presence of internal echoes or cul-de-sac fluid.
D. B and C

12. Identify the numbered structures shown in Figure 5-1.

1. ___   A. Vagina
2. ___   B. Urethra
3. ___   C. Pubic
              symphysis
4. ___   D. Posterior fornix
5. ___   E. Uterus
6. ___   F. Urinary bladder

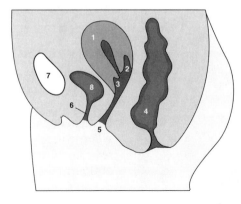

Figure 5-1. Female pelvis (sagittal view).

7. ___   G. Anterior fornix
8. ___   H. Rectum

13. The patient is a 9-year-old girl whose pelvic sonogram revealed the presence of multiple small cysts within the ovary. Considering her age, additional diagnostic tests are indicated to rule out:
A. diabetes.
B. polycystic kidney disease.
C. hypothyroidism.
D. adrenal dysfunction.

14. The normal position of the uterus is:
A. retroverted.
B. antiverted.
C. retroflexed.
D. antiflexed.

15. Using the most sensitive pregnancy tests, the presence of an intrauterine pregnancy can be detected as early as _____ days after ovulation.
A. 4–5
B. 7–10

C. 12–14

D. 16–21

16. The sonographic pattern of *in utero* infantile polycystic kidney disease is one of bilateral renal enlargement. Renal enlargement is demonstrated when the fetal kidney circumference exceeds _____ of the abdominal circumference.

A. 15%

B. 22%

C. 33%

D. 40%

17. Tubal pregnancies commonly rupture between _____ weeks of gestation.

A. 4–6

B. 6–8

C. 8–10

D. none of the above

18. The cell layer that expresses or determines the embryo's "masculinity" or "femininity" consists of:

A. strumal cells.

B. androgenic response cells.

C. primordial germ cells.

D. chordaea cells.

19. The endometrium is sonographically recognized as a hypoechoic region with a variable width. In its atrophic state, the endometrium will measure _____ , while in its secretory state the measurement is approximately _____ .

A. 1.5 mm; 9 mm

B. 1–2 mm; 7 mm

C. 1–3 mm; 5–7 mm

D. 2.5 mm; 11 mm

20. Identify the numbered structures shown in Figure 5-2.

1. ___   A. Allantois
2. ___   B. Amnion
3. ___   C. Chorion
4. ___   D. Extraembryonic coelom
5. ___   E. Embryo
6. ___   F. Yolk sac

21. Normal fetal heart rates are generally _____ beats per minute.

A. 100–120

B. 120–140

C. 120–160

D. 160–200

22. Congenital cervical incompetence is one of the complications associated with *in utero* exposure to:

A. environmental toxins.

B. diethylstilbestrol.

C. inadequate maternal nutrition.

D. placental abruption.

23. The fetal urinary bladder should routinely be sono-

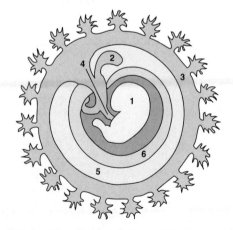

Figure 5-2. Six weeks' gestation.

graphically visible at approx-
imately _____ weeks of ges-
tation.
A. 9–10
B. 12–14
C. 14–15
D. 16–18

24. The sonographic characteristic
of a meningocele is:
A. a herniated sac protruding
from an area along the spinal column.
B. an encapsulated lesion
located along the spinal
column.
C. an open spinal defect.
D. the presence of strands of
neural tissue within a herniated sac protruding from
the spine.

25. In pregnant women the hCG
level will double approximately:
A. every day.
B. every other day.
C. every two days.
D. every three days.

26. The exclusion of fetal ven-
triculomegaly is best ac-
complished by sonographic
measurement of the:
A. choroid plexus.
B. ambient cisterns.
C. lateral ventricular atria.
D. caudate nucleus.

27. The growth of fibroids coexist-
ing with an intrauterine preg-
nancy is stimulated by:
A. estrogen.
B. progesterone.
C. hCG.
D. increased vascularity.

28. It is important to obtain precise measurements of any
pathology discovered in association with pregnancy to determine if any possible change in
size or structure occurs during
the pregnancy. Of the following
entities, which one tends to increase in size throughout the
duration of pregnancy?
A. Corpus luteum cysts
B. Follicular cysts
C. Cystadenomas
D. Graafian follicles

29. Which of the following statements about amniotic sheets
is *untrue?*
A. Composed of 1 layer of amniochorionic membrane
B. Composed of 2 layers of
amniochorionic membrane
C. Have a triangular base and
thickened free edge
D. Are not associated with increased risk of fetal anomalies but may restrict fetal
motion

30. What is the significance of the
"double bubble" sign?
A. Dilated proximal
duodenum
B. Dilated CBD
C. Dilated antrum of the
stomach
D. A and C

31. Transperineal sonography is
indicated in cases of:
A. early labor.
B. cervical incompetence or
PROM.
C. placenta previa.
D. all of the above

Match the following structures with the correct definitions.

A. Rectus abdominus muscle
B. Obturator internus muscle
C. Pubococcygeus muscle
D. Fornices
E. Pubic symphysis
F. Coccygeus muscle
G. Vagina
H. Sacrum
I. Rectum
J. Levator ani muscle group

32. ___ A fibrocartilaginous union of the pubic bones

33. ___ Triangular muscle extending posteromedially along both side walls of the true pelvis, parallel and adjacent to the lateral pelvic wall

34. ___ Hammock-like muscle stretching from pubis to coccyx

35. ___ Most superior of three muscles forming the pelvic diaphragm

36. ___ Roughly triangular-shaped muscle; originates at sacrum, courses laterally through greater sciatic foramen; inserts on greater trochanter of the femur

37. ___ Part of the levator ani muscle group; only function is to provide support to the sacrum

38. ___ Curved triangular bone composed of 5 united vertebrae

39. ___ Lower part of intestine terminating in the anal canal

40. ___ Thin-walled muscular tube extending from uterine cervix to the vestibule of the external genitalia

41. ___ Arched surfaces of a cul-de-sac

42. The maximum size of a "dominant" follicle may reach:
A. 10 mm.
B. 1 cm.
C. 20 mm.
D. 4 cm.

43. Elevated msAFP is associated with all of the following pathologies *except:*
A. anencephaly.
B. trisomy 21.
C. twins.
D. chorioangioma.

44. In the postmenopausal woman, endometrial thickening greater than _____ is indicative of an endometrial abnormality.
A. 4 mm
B. 5 mm
C. 8 mm
D. 9 mm

45. The *tip of the iceberg* sign is associated with:
A. serous cystadenoma.
B. endometrioma.
C. dermoid cyst.
D. fibroma.

46. Which of the following statements concerning interstitial ectopic pregnancy is (are) *untrue?*

A. Associated with a later rupture stage than other tubal locations
B. Will demonstrate a myometrial mantle
C. Subject to rapid exsanguination following rupture
D. Inevitably requires surgical treatment

47. Sonographic demonstration of a gestational sac within the uterine cavity is expected by the time hCG levels reach:
A. 300–750 MIU/ml (2nd I.S.).
B. 1025 mIU/ml (IRP).
C. 1400–1800 mIU/ml (IRP).
D. A and B

48. The earliest sonographically identifiable structure within a gestational sac is the:
A. fetal pole.
B. primary yolk sac.
C. secondary yolk sac.
D. embryonic disc.

49. What sonographic signs differentiate a cystic hygroma from an encephalocele?
A. Its location
B. Presence of septations or lymphedema
C. Its size
D. B and C

50. Which of the following is *not* an indicator of Down's syndrome?
A. Nuchal thickening
B. Shortened femur and humerus
C. Low AFP levels
D. None of the above

51. What is the significance of the sonographic "crescent" sign?
A. Vanishing twin
B. Placenta previa
C. Subchorionic hemorrhage
D. Amniotic bands

52. The earliest that fetal heart rates can be detected with transvaginal techniques is approximately:
A. 5 weeks' LMP.
B. 6 weeks' LMP.
C. 7 weeks' LMP.
D. 8 weeks' LMP.

53. The distal femoral epiphyses are sonographically visible at approximately _____ weeks of menstrual age.
A. 26
B. 30
C. 33
D. 36

54. Alpha fetoprotein is initially produced in the _____ and later by the fetal liver.
A. allantois
B. yolk sac
C. amnion
D. chorion

55. Correct measurement of the nuchal fold requires:
A. a coronal fetal head scan demonstrating cavum, thalami, and falx.
B. measurement from the outer limit of the occipital bone to the skin edge.
C. fetal head scans demonstrating the cerebellum and brain stem.
D. B and C

56. The union of the sperm and ovum produces a single cell called a (an):
    A. morula.
    B. blastocyst.
    C. zygote.
    D. embryo.

57. A 42-year-old female presents with a diagnosis of large-for-gestational-age, to rule out possible twin pregnancy. Sonography demonstrates the presence of two intrauterine sacs. One sac contains a single live fetus, crown-rump length consistent with 9 weeks' gestation. An anterior placenta is seen adjacent to this sac. A second sac is seen to abut a grossly enlarged, inhomogeneous placenta. This second sac demonstrates no evidence of fetal echoes. No adnexal masses are noted. Based on the sonographic evidence, this most likely represents a:
    A. fetus and partial mole.
    B. coexisting fetus and mole.
    C. single pregnancy and degenerating fibroid.
    D. partial mole.

58. Omphalocele may exist as an isolated anomaly or in association with other major malformations. Omphalocele has been noted in all of the following severe anomaly groups *except:*
    A. trisomy syndromes.
    B. pentalogy of Cantrell.
    C. Klinefelter syndrome.
    D. cloacal exstrophy.

59. Absence of cardiac activity in embryos greater than or equal to _____ mm is reliably associated with embryonic demise.
    A. 3
    B. 4
    C. 5
    D. 6

60. During the course of a fetal survey, if the sonographer is unable to demonstrate the fetal urinary bladder, it is important to rescan that area in approximately:
    A. 5–10 minutes.
    B. 15–45 minutes.
    C. 2 hours.
    D. 24 hours.

61. A vein of Galen malformation will demonstrate the following sonographic characteristics:
    A. oval- or cigar-shaped aneurysm.
    B. accompanying heterogeneous cystic areas.
    C. fused thalami.
    D. A and B

62. Twin embolization syndrome is associated with:
    A. monochorionic twins.
    B. "disappearing" twin syndrome.
    C. dichorionic twins.
    D. heterogeneous ectopic pregnancy.

63. Heart defects that can be missed by omitting evaluation of the outflow tracts are:
    A. tetralogy of Fallot.
    B. pentalogy of Cantrell.

C. Ebstein's anomaly.

D. A and B

64. When an incompetent cervix is diagnosed early in a pregnancy, a cervical _____ may be used to help sustain the pregnancy.
    A. diaphragm
    B. pessary
    C. cervical cerclage
    D. insertion of a mucous plug

65. The portion of the fallopian tube closest to the ovary is the:
    A. ampullary.
    B. infundibular.
    C. fimbriae.
    D. interstitial.

66. Fetal exposure to DES may lead to the development of a:
    A. didelphic uterus.
    B. T-shaped uterus.
    C. retroverted uterus.
    D. incarcerated uterus.

67. Sonographic demonstration of a fetus with an occipital encephalocele, multicystic kidneys, and polydactyly is typical of _____ syndrome.
    A. Turner's
    B. Kleebattschädel
    C. Meckel's
    D. Noonan's

68. When measuring the femur it is important to:
    A. measure both femurs and average the results.
    B. select the femur closest to the transducer.
    C. select the femur most distal to the transducer.

D. measure only symmetrical femurs.

69. The sides of the vaginal walls are enclosed by the:
    A. piriformis muscles.
    B. levator ani muscles.
    C. obturator muscles.
    D. psoas muscles.

70. Select the following pathologies in descending order of malignancy resulting in patient mortality.
    A. Endometrial, ovarian, cervical
    B. Endometrial, cervical, ovarian
    C. Ovarian, cervical, endometrial
    D. Ovarian, endometrial, cervical

71. Identify the numbered structures shown in Figure 5-3.

    1. ___   A. Amniotic cavity
    2. ___   B. Amnion

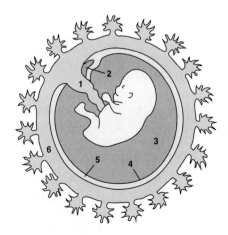

Figure 5-3. Eight weeks' gestation.

3. ___   C. Extraembryonic
            coelom
4. ___   D. Umbilical cord
5. ___   E. Chorion
6. ___   F. Yolk sac

72. Papillary projections seen within an adnexal mass have been associated with:
    A. intratumoral adhesions.
    B. a benign process within the tumor.
    C. a potentially malignant process within the tumor.
    D. fat within the tumor.

73. Histologically, the uterus consists of three tissue layers: perimetrium, myometrium, and endometrium. The perimetrial layer is also known as the ___ layer, and the endometrial layer is also known as the ___ layer.
    A. mucous; serous
    B. muscular; serous
    C. serous; mucous
    D. membranous; striated

74. Whenever uterine anomalies are found sonographers should also scan the ___ for associated anomalies.
    A. liver
    B. pancreas
    C. kidneys
    D. spleen

75. Follicular development and ovulation are stimulated by:
    A. estrogen.
    B. FSH and LH.
    C. progesterone.
    D. hCG.

76. The term ___ describes the developmental stage of the products of conception during implantation within the uterus.
    A. *morula*
    B. *ovum*
    C. *blastocyst*
    D. *trophoblast*

77. A predisposing condition associated with the development of uterine synechiae is:
    A. previous curettage or C-section.
    B. congenital uterine anomalies.
    C. DES exposure.
    D. chronic endometritis.

78. In which portion of the fallopian tube are ectopic pregnancies most likely to attach?
    A. Fimbriae
    B. Ampulla
    C. Interstitial
    D. Isthmus

79. Monochorionic twin pregnancies will include all of the following sonographic signs *except:*
    A. continuous adjacent placentae.
    B. gender differences.
    C. thin septal membranes.
    D. discordant fetal growth.

80. Failure of the embryonic kidney to ascend into the abdomen results in a pelvic ectopic kidney. Such a kidney takes its blood supply from any of the following *except:*

A. the inferior end of the aorta.
B. the iliac artery.
C. the medial sacral artery.
D. the renal artery.

81. During pregnancy, it is normal to observe an increase in gallbladder volume; therefore, the normal caliber of the common duct during pregnancy will:
    A. increase.
    B. decrease.
    C. vary.
    D. remain unchanged.

82. Color Doppler imaging has been found to improve the detection of malignant ovarian masses by demonstrating:
    A. an increased PI.
    B. pulsatile indices <1.
    C. decreased peripheral vascularity.
    D. A and C

83. Large for gestational age (LGA) fetuses are at greater risk for all of the following *except:*
    A. PROM.
    B. shoulder dystocia and birth trauma.
    C. meconium aspiration.
    D. prolonged labor.

84. Renal anomalies associated with trisomy 13 include:
    A. hyperlobulation.
    B. dysplasia and cortical cysts.
    C. renal agenesis.
    D. A and B

85. The area(s) of greatest clinical application of Doppler ultrasound to fetal studies is (are):

A. IUGR and twin gestation.
B. pregnancies complicated by infection.
C. suspected placenta previa.
D. all of the above

86. A Gartner's duct cyst shares a similar sonographic pattern with:
    A. abscess.
    B. cervical ectopic pregnancy.
    C. choreocarcinoma.
    D. adenomyosis.

87. Identify the numbered anatomical structures shown in Figure 5-4.

1. ___	A. Peritoneum
2. ___	B. Uterus
3. ___	C. External iliac artery
4. ___	D. Illiopsoas
5. ___	E. Obturator internis muscle
6. ___	F. Ovary
7. ___	G. External iliac vein

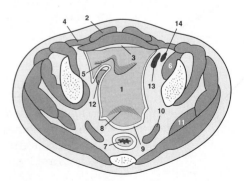

Figure 5-4. Female pelvis (sacral region).

8. ____   H. Rectus
                abdominus
                muscle

9. ____   I. Pouch of
                Douglas

10. ____   J. Piriformis
                muscle

11. ____   K. Fallopian tube

12. ____   L. Coccygeus
                muscle

13. ____   M. Peritoneal
                cavity

14. ____   N. Rectum

88. If the long axis of a fetal foot
and the tibia and fibula are
imaged in the same scan
plane, the most likely diagnosis is:
A. talipes equinovarus.
B. dwarfism.
C. club foot.
D. A and C

89. During embryogenesis, the am-
niotic cavity originates within
the _____ , while the primitive
yolk sac forms adjacent to the
_____ .
A. endoderm; ectoderm
B. ectoderm; endoderm
C. endoderm; mesoderm
D. ectoderm; mesoderm

90. A cleft palate is associated with
all of the following conditions
except:
A. Meckel-Gruber.
B. hypertelorism.
C. chromosomal
abnormalities.
D. erythroblastosis fetalis.

91. During a fetal cardiac survey,
movement of the flap of the foramen ovale should be documented. The foramen ovale is
located within the:
A. right atrium.
B. left atrium.
C. right ventricle.
D. left ventricle.

92. Fetal intracranial calcifications
are commonly associated with:
A. viral infections.
B. hemoglobinopathies.
C. diabetic pregnancies.
D. IUGR.

93. What ovarian sonographic patterns should a sonographer ex-
pect to see in a young woman
in her mid-twenties with a four
year history of oral contraceptive use?
A. Multiple follicular cysts and
a dominant follicle
B. Theca lutein cysts
C. Atretic, irregular follicular
cysts
D. Nonfunctioning ovary

94. With persistent truncus arte-
riosus, a large _____ defect is
usually present.
A. atrial septal defect
B. ventricular septal defect
C. mitral stenosis
D. tricuspid stenosis

95. In a 4-year-old patient presenting with vaginal bleeding the
sonographer should be alert to
the possibility of:
A. hematocolpos, hema-
tometra, hemosalpinx.
B. sarcoma botryoides or uterine adenocarcinoma.

C. a foreign object within the
   vagina.
D. B and C

96. Reverberation and multipath
    reflections are two artifacts as-
    sociated with scanning a full
    urinary bladder. Such artifacts
    may be avoided by:
    A. raising the system gain.
    B. partial emptying of the
       bladder.
    C. repositioning transducer or
       scanning angle.
    D. B and C

97. The acronym *GIFT* stands for:
    A. gammete intrafallopian
       transfer.
    B. gonadal *in vitro* fertilization
       therapy.
    C. gynecologic *in vitro*
       fertilization technique.
    D. A and C

98. Spina bifida may be classified
    as:
    A. spina bifida occulta.
    B. spina bifida Arnold-Chiari.
    C. spina bifida cystica.
    D. A and C

99. Which of the following sonolu-
    cent structures are most fre-
    quently observed within the
    fetal abdomen?
    A. Stomach; kidney; gall-
       bladder
    B. Aorta; gallbladder; kidney
    C. Stomach; aorta; urinary
       bladder
    D. Jrinary bladder; kidney;
       stomach

100. During pregnancy, a corpus
     luteum cyst should regress by
     approximately _____ weeks.
     A. 9–10
     B. 10–12
     C. 14–15
     D. 16–20

101. Which of the following state-
     ments concerning fetal lung
     maturity is *incorrect*?
     A. Maturity corresponds with
        an L/S ratio of 2 or greater
     B. Maternal diabetes mellitus
        is associated with delayed
        lung maturity
     C. L/S stands for lecithin/sur-
        factant
     D. Chronic maternal hyper-
        tension may accelerate
        fetal lung maturity

102. When obtaining umbilical ar-
     tery waveforms, the pregnant
     patient should be placed in
     the _____ position.
     A. semi-recumbent, with a
        right lateral tilt
     B. semi-recumbent, with left
        lateral tilt
     C. right lateral decubitus
     D. left lateral decubitus

103. Echoes returning from struc-
     tures distal to a cyst appear
     as high-amplitude structures
     on the screen. This condition
     is produced by the following
     artifact:
     A. beam divergence.
     B. slice thickness.
     C. mirror image.
     D. acoustic enhancement.

104. A 21-year-old primagravida with third-trimester bleeding was sent to ultrasound. A very large, complexly echogenic mass was unexpectedly discovered posterior to the sacrum. What appeared to be calcium deposits within the mass showed evidence of acoustic shadowing. The most likely diagnosis in this case is:
    A. Ascherman's syndrome.
    B. spina bifida.
    C. sacral coccygeal teratoma.
    D. meningomyelocele.

105. Superficial body-wall trauma is most often implicated in hemorrhage into the:
    A. pouch of Douglas.
    B. anterior cul-de-sac.
    C. space of Retzius.
    D. utero-vesicular space.

106. Which of the following statements concerning cleft lip is *untrue*?
    A. Oblique coronal views are recommended
    B. May be isolated or associated with major anomalies
    C. Make observation when lips are closed
    D. Make observation when lips are open

107. The patient was a 20-year-old gravida 1 para 0 female, sent to rule out SGA fetus. Ultrasound studies revealed the presence of a hypoechoic region in the fundal portion of the placenta which displayed random motion. No Doppler signal was obtained from the region. The area is very near the placental insertion of the umbilical cord and measures approximately 2.8 × 2.2 cm. No other abnormalities of the placenta were identified. The differential diagnosis in this case is:
    A. venous lake.
    B. placental abruption.
    C. early chorioangioma.
    D. A or C

108. A sign or symptom of pre-eclampsia is:
    A. hypertension with proteinuria.
    B. marked edema.
    C. convulsions.
    D. A and B

109. Grade III placentae are found in _____ of term pregnancies.
    A. 5%
    B. 10%–20%
    C. 30%
    D. 1/3

110. Gastroschisis can be differentiated from omphalocele by demonstrating:
    A. free-floating viscera.
    B. presence of the umbilical cord remote from the defect.
    C. presence of the cord entering the apex of the defect.
    D. A and B

111. A 16-year-old primigravid female was referred to the ultrasound department for estimation of fetal age. A single

fetus showing signs of fetal edema, abdominal ascites, and both pericardial and pleural effusions was demonstrated. Amniotic fluid volume was severely decreased. Fetal kidneys and bladder, however, were visualized. The presence of the three abnormal fetal fluid collections suggests the presence of:
A. cystic hygroma.
B. anasarca.
C. Grebe's disease.
D. B and C

112. Fetal pelviectasis of not more than _____ mm is considered to be normal physiologic dilatation.
A. 3
B. 6
C. 9
D. 11

113. Which of the following statements concerning chorioangioma is *untrue?*
A. Represents a severe form of amniotic band syndrome
B. Represents a placental neoplasm
C. Is associated with elevated alpha fetoprotein
D. May cause fetal asphyxiation

114. Ultrasound of the postpartum uterus is effective in ruling out the presence of clinically significant retained placental tissue when the following pattern(s) is (are) demonstrated.
A. Isolated endometrial fluid

B. Uninterrupted central cavity echo
C. Hyperechoic foci without an associated mass
D. All of the above

115. Abruptio placentae is usually diagnosed clinically and confirmed at delivery. However, at times an abruption may be visualized sonographically. Based on the appearance of the sonographic patterns alone, the following differential diagnoses must be considered.
A. Hydatidiform mole
B. Chorioangioma
C. Engorged myometrial veins
D. All of the above

116. A 45-year-old, nulligravid patient was referred for pelvic sonography to evaluate complaints of "pressure" and a dull ache in the lower pelvic region. Scans demonstrated a retroverted uterus filling the cul-de-sac. Multiple indentations of the bladder wall were seen wherever it contacted the uterine structure. Posterior sound transmission was unsatisfactory. These findings are suggestive of:
A. endometriosis.
B. leiomyoma.
C. uterine incarceration.
D. congenital uterine anomaly.

117. Toxemia of pregnancy is characterized by hypertension (with or without proteinuria).

The condition generally occurs in the _____ trimester of pregnancy.
A. first
B. second
C. third
D. A and B

118. A form of endometriosis which results in endometrial tissue invasion of the myometrium and diffuse uterine enlargement is called:
A. adenomyomatosis.
B. endometrial hyperplasia.
C. adenomyosis.
D. endometrial polyps.

119. The cisterna magna should be measured between the _____ and the _____ .
A. vermis; fourth ventricle
B. vermis; occipital bone
C. peduncles; fourth ventricle
D. peduncles; sylvian fissure

120. When two or more embryologically unrelated anomalies occur together at a higher than expected rate, they constitute a:
A. sequence.
B. syndrome.
C. disorder.
D. disaster.

121. What is the most frequent cause of congenital hydrocephaly?
A. Aqueductal stenosis
B. Holoprosencephaly
C. Spina bifida
D. Ventriculomegaly

122. Omphaloceles containing only bowel are associated with:
A. bowel obstructions.
B. underlying chromosomal disorders.
C. meconium ileus.
D. A and C

123. A patient referred to ultrasound to evaluate the presence or absence of her IUCD admits that she voided just before entering the department because her full bladder was too uncomfortable. What special steps, if any, should the sonographer carry out?
A. Scold the patient and send her home
B. Tell the referring physician
C. Rehydrate the patient and wait 20 minutes before performing the scan
D. Use a lower-frequency transducer to achieve adequate penetration

124. In a scan to rule out placenta previa, if the fetal head obstructs complete visualization of the distal edge of a placenta the sonographer should:
A. measure the distance between the fetal skull and the maternal sacral promontory.
B. place the patient in trendelenburg position.
C. try translabial or transperineal scanning.
D. all of the above

125. The sonographic diagnosis of an embryonic pregnancy should be considered in the presence of:
    A. an abnormally large sac (>25 mm) that lacks an embryo.
    B. a gestational sac (>20 mm) that lacks a yolk sac.
    C. a gestational sac without evidence of decidual activity.
    D. A and B

126. Second trimester sonographic demonstration of frontal bone angulation with or without hydrocephaly denotes the:
    A. halo sign.
    B. banana sign.
    C. lemon sign.
    D. Spalding's sign.

127. Placental size can be an indicator of pregnancy complication. After 23 weeks, placental enlargement is suspected in a placenta thicker than _____ cm; in contrast, an abnormally thin placenta is one that measures less than _____ cm.
    A. 4; 2
    B. 5; 1.5
    C. 6; 1
    D. 7; 3

128. Fusion of the amnion and the chorion is expected to occur by:
    A. 10 weeks.
    B. 12 weeks.
    C. 14 weeks.
    D. 16 weeks.

129. Intrauterine growth retardation (IUGR) can be divided into two types:
    A. symmetrical and asymmetrical.
    B. intrinsic and extrinsic.
    C. second and third trimester.
    D. A and B

Match the following definitions to the numbered terms.
    A. Same gene received from each parent
    B. Hereditary factors (DNA)
    C. Any nonsex chromosome
    D. Microscopic rod-shaped bodies
    E. Different type gene for a particular trait received from each parent

130. ____ Autosome

131. ____ Chromosomes

132. ____ Genes

133. ____ Homozygous

134. ____ Heterozygous

135. Which of the following statements concerning cystic teratoma is *untrue*?
    A. Anechoic cystic teratomas tend to occur in young girls
    B. Sebum within a dermoid may collect anteriorly
    C. Cystic teratoma is classified as a physiologic cyst

D. The incidence of peritonitis increases with rup-
ture

136. The sonographic demonstration of a prominent hypo-
echoic area within the posterior aspect of the early
developing fetal brain represents the:
A. rhombencephalon.
B. trelencephalon.
C. tentorium.
D. caudate nucleus.

137. Cervical length in healthy
pregnancy normally ranges
from _____ to _____ cm.
A. 2.0; 4.0
B. 2.5; 5.0
C. 3.5; 6.0
D. 4.0; 6.5

138. The point of origin of the fal-
lopian tube is the:
A. isthmus.
B. ampulla.
C. fimbria.
D. uterine cornu.

139. In monochorionic pregnancies, the absence of a separating amniotic membrane
should prompt a sonographer
to search for possible:
A. asymmetrical growth.
B. polyhydramnios.
C. conjoined twins.
D. all of the above

140. Idiopathic polyhydramnios is
most common during weeks
_____ to _____ of pregnancy.
A. 18; 24
B. 20; 30

C. 24; 32
D. 28; 34

141. Stein-Leventhal syndrome is
often associated with all of
the following *except:*
A. hirsutism.
B. menorrhagia.
C. infertility.
D. bilaterally enlarged
ovaries.

142. A low head-abdomen ratio
should raise the questions of:
A. macrocephaly.
B. microcephaly.
C. macrosomia.
D. B and C

143. When a patient is referred for
evaluation of a fetus small for
gestational age (SGA), the following conditions should be
considered:
A. incorrect dates or unusual
fetal lie.
B. oligohydramnios, IUGR.
C. erythroblastosis fetalis.
D. A and B

144. All of the following statements
concerning crown-rump
length measurements are
true *except:*
A. inaccurate 10 weeks (post
conception)
B. inaccurate if longest axis
of the fetus is not chosen
for measurement
C. best measured between 6
to 12 weeks (LMP)
D. is the optimal method of
establishing fetal age

145. Which of the following is *not*

recommended for disinfecting transvaginal transducers?
A. Sporicidin
B. Cidex
C. Autoclaving
D. Diluted bleach

146. Characteristic(s) of Meigs' syndrome is (are):
A. hydrothorax and ascites.
B. pelvic mass (usually ovarian fibroma).
C. resolution of syndrome after tumor removal.
D. all of the above

147. Acute pelvic inflammatory disease (PID) typically produces all of the following *except:*
A. loss of tissue planes or margins.
B. thick-walled, echogenic fluid collections.
C. thin-walled, echo-free fluid collections.
D. A and C

148. During obstetrical scanning, if the patient complains of feeling faint and nauseated, the sonographer should:
A. open a window.
B. scan faster.
C. turn the patient on her left side.
D. turn the patient on her right side.

149. The optimal instrument setting for sonographic evaluation of an intrauterine contraceptive device (IUD) is:
A. higher gain.
B. lower gain.

C. increased time gain compensation.
D. increased slope start.

150. The most common site(s) of metastatic lesions from pelvic masses is (are):
A. para-aortic nodes.
B. peritoneum.
C. liver.
D. all of the above

151. The sonographic pattern(s) of pseudocyesis is (are):
A. misshapen gestational sac.
B. evidence of a pseudogestational sac.
C. evidence of a blighted ovum.
D. none of the above

152. A patient referred to the ultrasound department from the OB clinic has been described as a G4P1012. This simplified method of expressing a patient's reproductive history indicates that the patient has had:
A. 2 live children.
B. 3 live children.
C. 4 pregnancies.
D. A and C

153. Two normal variants in fetal head shape may be seen in the third trimester. A short, wide fetal head is referred to as _____ ; an elongated, flattened head is referred to as _____ .
A. brachycephaly; dolicocephaly
B. macrocephaly; microcephaly

C. dolicocephaly; brachy-
cephaly

D. microcephaly; macro-
cephaly

154. The fetal vein that connects
the umbilical vein to the IVC
and runs obliquely through
the liver is the:
A. left portal vein.
B. ductus venosum.
C. ductus venosus.
D. right portal vein.

155. Which of the following ovarian
tumors are associated with
changes in a patient's secondary sex characteristics?
A. Arrhenoblastoma and
granulosa cell
B. Dysgerminoma and
Brenner
C. Serous and mucinous
cystadenoma
D. Fibroma and Krukenberg
tumors

156. The growth of the gestational
sac in normal pregnancy is
approximately:
A. 0.5–1 mm/day; 2 cm/wk.
B. 1–1.1 mm/day; 3.5 cm/wk.
C. 2–2.5 mm/day; 4 cm/wk.
D. none of the above

157. Which of the following statements concerning tubo-ovarian abscesses is *untrue*?
A. Usually unilateral
B. Usually bilateral
C. Produces thick-walled,
irregularly shaped struc-
tures
D. May demonstrate internal
fluid-fluid levels

158. Risk factors associated with
the development of placental
abruptions include a previous
history of abruption and:
A. trauma.
B. cocaine abuse or cigarette
smoking.
C. congenital uterine
anomalies.
D. all of the above

159. During sonography of a
7-week pregnancy, a well-
shaped gestational sac containing a yolk sac and embryonic pole was seen. The sac
and contents appeared com-
patible with dates, and filled
the endometrial cavity except
for a small, crescent-shaped
lucency between the fundus
and the superior edge of the
sac. The patient denied experiencing any spotting, bleeding, or cramping. The sonolucent "space" most likely
represents:
A. the double gestational sac
sign.
B. chorioamnion separation.
C. implantation bleeding.
D. an elevated chorion.

160. Oligohydramnios, the dimin-
ishment in the amount of
amniotic fluid during pregnancy, sends a strong diagnostic signal. Oligohydramnios is most often associated
with which of the following
conditions?
A. IUGR and duodenal
atresia
B. Postmaturity and Potter's
syndrome

C. IPKD

D. Chorioangioma

161. List the three types of breech presentation in their descending order of incidence:
    A. frank, footling, and complete.
    B. complete, frank and footling.
    C. frank, complete, and footling.
    D. complete, footling, and frank.

162. An aid in evaluating fetal position is present in the appearance of the thalamus. The _____ of the thalamus always points to the fetal spine.
    A. base
    B. flare
    C. apex
    D. A and B

163. Which of the following statements concerning Rh sensitization is *untrue?*
    A. Can be prevented with RhoGam immunization within 4 days of delivery of an Rh-positive fetus
    B. RhoGam must be administered after every Rh-positive delivery
    C. RhoGam is often routinely given to Rh-negative gravidas after 20 weeks
    D. Fetal effects may include hepatosplenomegaly

164. The pregnant endometrium is composed of the decidua:
    A. capsularis, vera, basale.

B. capsularis, parietalis, basalis.
C. basalis, compactum, vera.
D. capsularis, basale, spongiosum.

Irregularities in placental size or echogenicity occur with specific pregnancy complications or abnormal conditions. Match the following placental descriptions to the numbered list of pregnancy complications or abnormalities. The descriptions can be used more than once.
    A. increased placental size and thickness
    B. decreased placental size and thickness
    C. sonolucencies within the placenta
    D. calcifications within the placenta

165. ___ pregnancy induced hypertension

166. ___ fetal cardiac disease

167. ___ maternal renal disease

168. ___ maternal diabetes

169. ___ intrauterine growth retardation

170. ___ preeclampsia

171. ___ maternal Rh isoimmunization

172. ___ maternal syphilis

173. ___ placental infarcts

174. ___ chorioangioma

175. Congenital cystic adenoma-toid malformation (CAM) Type II results in bilateral thin-wal-led, small cysts (<1 cm) within the upper pole of the fetal lung. This condition is associated with:
    A. renal agenesis and prune belly syndrome.
    B. diaphragmatic hernia.
    C. pulmonary sequestration.
    D. lymphangioma or heman-gioma.

176. Biparietal diameter (BPD) measurements are most ac-curate (to within ± 1 wk) at approximately _____ weeks' gestation; accuracy of the BPD diminishes (± 2–4 weeks' gestation) after _____ weeks.
    A. 16; 32
    B. 18; 34
    C. 20; 36
    D. 22; 38

177. The use of _____ and _____ increase the user's risk for ec-topic pregnancy.
    A. antibiotics; tampons
    B. danacrin; tubal insuffla-tion techniques
    C. fertility drugs; oral con-traceptives
    D. none of the above

178. Pre-amniocentesis scans should locate:
    A. the fetus and placenta.
    B. the cord and maternal bladder.
    C. a suitable pocket of fluid.
    D. all of the above

179. The average gestational age for the incidence of a grade III placenta in normal pregnancy is:
    A. 35.5 weeks.
    B. 36.6 weeks.
    C. 37.0 weeks.
    D. 38.0 weeks.

180. The type of fibroid that is most likely to be mistaken for an adnexal mass is the _____ fibroid.
    A. degenerating
    B. calcified
    C. pedunculated
    D. hydropic

181. Theca lutein ovarian cysts are seen:
    A. with molar pregnancies.
    B. with Perganol therapy.
    C. with oral contraceptive use.
    D. A and B

182. Chorionic villus sampling (CVS) is usually performed at _____ gestation, with prelim-inary results available as early as _____ .
    A. 6–7 weeks; 24 hours
    B. 8–12 weeks; 48 hours
    C. 40th day; 12–20 hours
    D. 60th day; 8–16 hours

183. When performing abdominal circumference measurements it is important to ensure that a true transverse axis of the fetal abdomen has been im-aged. This can be achieved by demonstrating a scan in which the _____ lie in the

same plane (directly opposite one another).
A. right portal vein and fetal spine
B. fluid-filled stomach and spine
C. intraabdominal umbilical vein and spine
D. aorta and spine

184. The double gestational sac sign is a valuable observation in confirming the presence of an early intrauterine pregnancy. The double linear reflections are made by the _____ and the _____ .
A. decidua basalis; decidua capsularis
B. decidua capsularis; decidua parietalis
C. decidua vera; decidua basalis
D. decidua vera; decidua parietalis

185. Microcephaly is defined in the fetus as a head circumference more than _____ standard deviations below the mean.
A. 1
B. 2
C. 3
D. 4

186. Failure to demonstrate the fetal stomach should raise suspicions of:
A. diaphragmatic hernia.
B. esophageal atresia.
C. duodenal atresia.
D. pyloric stenosis.

187. While scanning a 32-week fetus you note that the vessels of the umbilical cord are widely separated by a large sonolucency. What abnormalities should come to mind?
A. Urachal cyst
B. Allantoic cyst
C. Umbilical artery aneurysm
D. Excessive deposit of Wharton's jelly

188. On a pelvic scan, what sonographic characteristic can be used to differentiate the ureters from the internal iliac veins?
A. Their shape and diameter
B. Distal blunting
C. Their pathway
D. Proximal bifurcation

189. Which of the following intrauterine contraceptive devices produces a longitudinal sonographic pattern of five interrupted echoes of moderate to high amplitude?
A. Dalkon shield
B. Progestasert
C. Lippes Loop
D. Paraguard

190. Placenta accreta and its variants, placenta increta and placenta percreta, are an important type of placental disorder that can potentially result in maternal morbidity and even the risk of mortality. Which of the following is *not* a high risk for developing this condition?
A. History of prior or repeated C-section

B. Low posterior placenta
C. Presence of focal exophytic masses
D. Placenta previa

191. The diagnostic sign of a cloverleaf skull is associated with:
    A. osteogenesis imperfecta.
    B. achondrogenesis.
    C. thanatophoric dwarfism.
    D. caudal regression syndrome.

192. The high mortality rate associated with congenital diaphragmatic hernia relates to the effects of this abnormality on the:
    A. bowel.
    B. heart.
    C. lung.
    D. stomach.

193. When a single umbilical artery is demonstrated on a fetal scan, sonographers should be alert to the possibility of:
    A. multiple malformations.
    B. additional anomalies.
    C. chromosomal disorders.
    D. all of the above

194. Select the *false* statement(s) about urinary bladder exstrophy.
    A. The bladder appears greatly distended
    B. Amniotic fluid volume is normal
    C. The defect involves the lower abdominal and anterior bladder walls
    D. All of the above

195. If the width of the cervix or uterus is more than 5 cm, the possibility of _____ must be explored.
    A. Rokitansky-Kuster-Hauser syndrome
    B. didelphic uterus
    C. bicornuate uterus
    D. subseptate uterus

196. Select the *false* statement regarding duodenal atresia.
    A. Associated trisomy 21 is present in ¹/₃ of cases
    B. Absence of peristalsis results from bowel obstruction
    C. May stem from the presence of an annular pancreas
    D. Polyhydramnios results from reduced amniotic fluid ingestion

197. Hydroureter is *not* an expected finding in which of the following conditions?
    A. Posterior urethral valve syndrome (PUVS)
    B. Ureteropelvic junction obstruction (UPJ)
    C. Ureterovesicular junction obstruction (UVJ)
    D. None of the above

198. The amniotic fluid index (AFI) has proven valuable in predicting the presence of polyhydramnios or oligohydramnios. A normal AFI is the sum of _____ in total vertical height of all four uterine quadrants.
    A. 4 cm

B. 8 cm
C. 16 cm
D. 24 cm

199. Abnormal enlargement of the fetal kidneys is associated with multicystic, polycystic, and dysplastic kidney disease as well as with:
A. Beckwith-Wiedeman syndrome and renal vein thrombosis.
B. Klinefelter syndrome.
C. Turner's syndrome.
D. Ascherman's syndrome.

200. When a comparison is made between fetal heart rate and maternal heart rate the fetal rate is usually:
A. ½ the maternal rate.
B. twice the maternal rate.
C. three times faster than the maternal rate.
D. quadruple the maternal rate.

201. A helpful technique in distinguishing the presence of

prune belly syndrome in a fetus with ascites is:
A. applying a stand-off device to the maternal wall.
B. tapping on the maternal abdominal wall.
C. high gain studies.
D. low gain studies.

202. The serum alpha fetoprotein test is most accurate at approximately _____ weeks of gestation.
A. 9
B. 11
C. 13
D. 15

203. Select the *false* statement(s) concerning chronic ectopic pregnancy.
A. Causes abdominal pain and associated low-grade fever
B. Represents a form of abdominal pregnancy
C. Caused by gradual disintegration of the tubal wall
D. A and C

CASES AND QUESTIONS

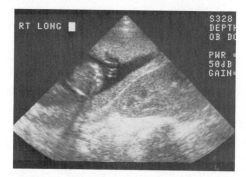

A

B

Figure 5-5. (A) Longitudinal scan slightly right of midline. (B) Transverse scan. (Courtesy of Patricia Lucas, Sinai Hospital, Baltimore, Maryland.)

The patient, a young gravid female, was referred for routine sonography to estimate fetal age.

204. During the course of the ultrasound study, the patient stated that her doctor had palpated a pelvic mass and suspected the presence of an ovarian cyst. Figure 5-5A, B demonstrates sonographic evidence of a (an):
   A. enlarged corpus luteum cyst.
   B. uterine fibroid.
   C. ectopic pregnancy.
   D. pelvic kidney.

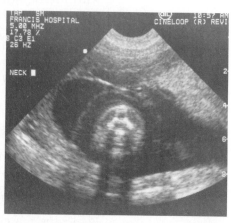

A

B

Figure 5-6. (A) Sagittal obstetrical scan. (B) Corresponding transverse scan. (Courtesy of Dayna Landru and Tracy Pfizenmaier, St. Francis Hospital School of Diagnostic Medical Sonography, Milwaukee, Wisconsin.)

Routine obstetrical sonogram to check "dates" on a G2P0AB1 female at approximately 24 weeks' gestation.

205. The images in Figure 5-6 demonstrate signs of the following pathology:
    A. cystic hygroma.
    B. encephalocele.
    C. nuchal cord.
    D. nuchal thickening.

transabdominal and transvaginal sonography was ordered.

206. Figure 5-7 demonstrates the presence of a (an):
    A. hemorrhagic corpus luteum cyst.
    B. ectopic pregnancy.
    C. endometrioma.
    D. blighted ovum.

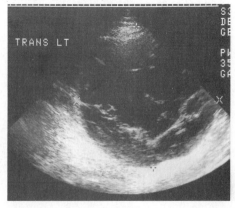

Figure 5-8. Transverse scan at the level of the uterine fundus and approximately 8 cm left of midline. (Courtesy of Stephanie Ellingson, University of Iowa Hospitals and Clinics, Iowa City, Iowa.)

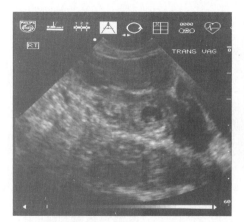

Figure 5-7. Transvaginal pelvic scan (transverse plane). (Courtesy of Lisa Elbert, Community College of Allegheny County, Monroeville, Pennsylvania.)

Figure 5-7 is a representative film from a study on a 22-year-old female with elevated hCG levels (3472 mIU/ml). Patient denied bleeding or pain. Three days prior to this study the patient underwent transabdominal ultrasound which was negative for either intrauterine pregnancy or adnexal masses. Because of increasing hCG levels and a past history of hysterosalpingogram diagnosis of a blocked left fallopian tube, repeat

A 28-year-old female is referred to your department at approximately 25 weeks' gestation to rule out anomalies, following ultrasound examination at another institution.

207. Which of the following best describes the sonographic findings in Figure 5-8?
    A. A simple cyst is seen adjacent to the uterine fundus
    B. A complex mass—primar-

ily cystic, but with septations—is seen adjacent to
the uterine fundus

C. Septations are seen within
the maternal bladder

D. A subchorionic fluid collection with internal septations is present in the
fundal region of the
uterus

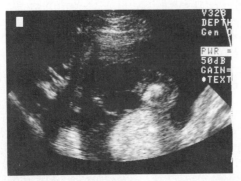

A

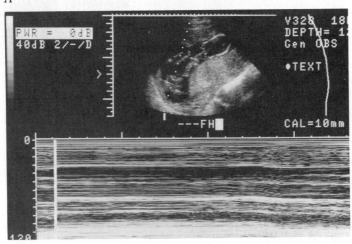

B

Figure 5-9. (A) Transverse scan of fetal skull. (B) Combined
M-mode and B-mode cardiac scans. (Courtesy of Janice St. Jean,
Rhode Island Hospital School of Diagnostic Ultrasound, Women
and Infants Hospital, Providence, Rhode Island.)

This patient presented for pre-amniocentesis sonography due to advanced maternal age. She had no family history of prior congenital anomalies. A single intrauterine gestation was demonstrated which measured 14.6 weeks, about 2 weeks behind dates by LMP.

208. Based on the findings in Figure 5-9, what is the most likely diagnosis?
   A. Teratoma
   B. Occipital cephalocele
   C. Cystic hygroma
   D. Meningomyelocele

209. In 80% of cases this condition involves the:
   A. head.
   B. neck.
   C. thorax.
   D. abdomen.

210. Which of the following conditions is associated with this abnormality?
   A. Lymphedema
   B. Neural tube defect
   C. Choroid plexus cysts
   D. Goiters

211. This defect is highly associated with the chromosomal abnormality:
   A. trisomy 21.
   B. trisomy 18.
   C. trisomy 13.
   D. Turner's syndrome.

212. What is the significance of the diagnostic information contained in Figure 5-9B?
   A. Demonstration of ventricular septal defect
   B. Documents fetal breathing
   C. Negative cardiac activity
   D. Documents fetal arrhythmia

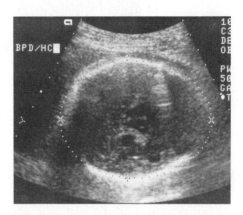

Figure 5-10. Transverse scan through fetal skull. (Courtesy of Linda Lang, Johns Hopkins School of Diagnostic Medical Sonography, Baltimore, Maryland.)

213. Figure 5-10 demonstrates a right ventricle measurement of 2.1 cm. Normal ventricular measurements after 16 weeks' gestation should be no greater than:
   A. 8 mm.
   B. 10 mm.
   C. 2 cm.
   D. 3 cm.

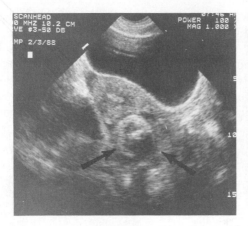

Figure 5-11. Sagittal scan of the female pelvis. (Courtesy of Benita Barthel, Ochsner Medical Foundation, New Orleans, Louisiana.)

The patient is a 25-year-old female with pelvic pain associated with nausea, weakness, and dizziness. She complains of dyspareunia for the past few months. Ultrasound of the pelvis was ordered.

214. The area depicted by arrows in Figure 5-11 is sonographically consistent with:
    A. endometrioma.
    B. fibroma.
    C. serous cystadenoma.
    D. cystic teratoma.

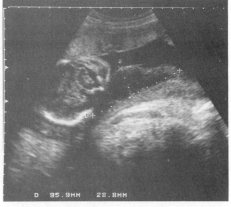

A

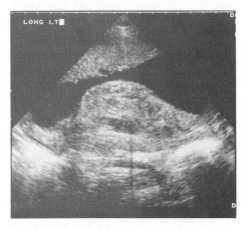

B

Figure 5-12. (A) Placental scan (19 weeks' gestation). (B) Placental scan (23 weeks' gestation). (Courtesy of Anita Bowser, Community College of Allegheny County, Monroeville, Pennsylvania.)

This 31-year-old patient presented with vaginal bleeding and mild abdominal cramping. The patient denied experiencing any recent trauma. Her first ultrasound examination demonstrated a placenta with an abnormal left posterior extension that seemed separate from the myometrium. Representative scans of her second (Fig. 5-12A) and third (Fig. 5-12B) ultrasound studies are presented here.

215. Based on the history and Figure 5-12A, what is the most likely diagnosis?
    A. Subamniotic hematoma
    B. Subchorionic hematoma
    C. Retroplacental abruption
    D. Preplacental abruption

216. Repeat scans taken at 23 weeks (Fig. 5-12B) again demonstrated the abnormal area; however, it had decreased in size and echogenicity. From its initial measurement of 10.3 cm × 7.7 cm × 3.3 cm to 3 cm × 2 cm × 1 cm. The marked decrease in size and shape of the "mass" can be explained on the basis of a:
    A. succenturiate lobe.
    B. fetus papyraceous.
    C. transient myometrial contraction.
    D. chorioangioma.

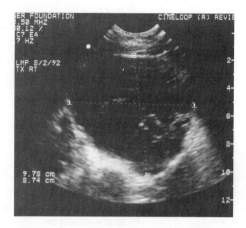

Figure 5-13. Transverse scan of the right adnexa. (Courtesy of Michelle Guillory, Ochsner Medical Foundation, New Orleans, Louisiana.)

This 30-year-old female complained of lower abdominal pain and distention. The patient was noted to have a pelvic mass during physical examination. Pelvic ultrasound (Fig. 5-13) was ordered today, 2 weeks since her last menstrual period.

217. The sonographic appearance of this adnexal mass is suggestive of:
    A. Stein-Leventhal syndrome.
    B. dermoid.
    C. mucinous cystadenoma.
    D. arrhenoblastoma.

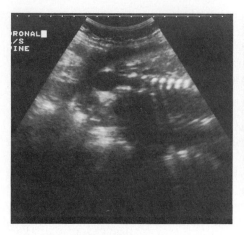

Figure 5-14. Scan of the fetal spine. (Courtesy of Bonnie S. Kazior, Community College of Allegheny County, Monroeville, Pennsylvania.)

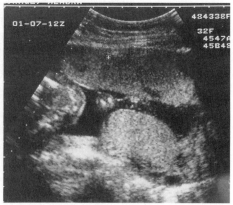

Figure 5-15. Second trimester longitudinal scan.

The patient was an elderly primigravida referred to evaluate fetal size and age in a pregnancy thought to be 29 weeks by dates. Sonography demonstrated a fetus in the cephalic position, at a gestational age of approximately 26 weeks. During the fetal survey an area of interest (Figure 5-14) was noted.

218. This scan demonstrates the presence of:
    A. sacral coccygeal teratoma.
    B. the fetal bladder.
    C. meningocele.
    D. cervical spina bifida.

This 23-year-old (gravida 2 para 1) female was referred to ultrasound for evaluation of vaginal bleeding.

219. Based on the appearance of the placenta in Figure 5-15, the most likely diagnosis is:
    A. placental abruption.
    B. complete previa.
    C. succenturiate placenta.
    D. senescent placenta.

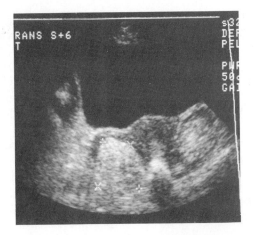

Figure 5-16. Longitudinal pelvic scan, approximately 3 cm right of midline. (Courtesy of Stephanie Ellingson, University of Iowa Hospitals and Clinics, Iowa City, Iowa.)

A 33-year-old female is referred to your ultrasound laboratory with complaints of chronic fatigue for the past two years. She has had menstrual irregularities since the onset of menses.

220. What are the ultra-sonographic findings demonstrated in Figure 5-16?
    A. Normal uterus with normal ovaries seen bilaterally
    B. Normal uterus with fluid-filled colon bilaterally
    C. Normal uterus and bilateral hyperechoic adnexal masses
    D. Abnormal uterus with bilateral hypoechoic adnexal masses

221. What additional techniques could the sonographer use to better characterize these findings?
    A. Perform a barium enema to delineate the bowel
    B. Perform a water enema to delineate the bowel
    C. Use a lower-frequency transducer to image with better detail
    D. Perform an air enema to help delineate the bowel

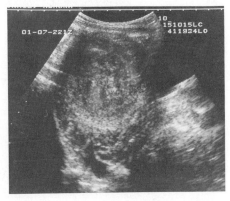

Figure 5-17. Longitudinal scan of the uterus.

A 42-year-old woman is referred to you for pelvic sonography to evaluate complaints of cramping pain during menstruation, frequency of urination, and constipation.

222. The longitudinal scan of the uterus seen in Figure 5-17 demonstrates sonographic evidence of:
    A. an endometrioma.
    B. a leiomyoma.
    C. trophoblastic disease.
    D. pelvic inflammatory disease.

223. What additional techniques would increase the specificity of the ultrasound diagnosis?
  A. Transabdominal scans
  B. Transperineal or translabial scans
  C. Water retention enema techniques
  D. Rescanning following a cleansing enema

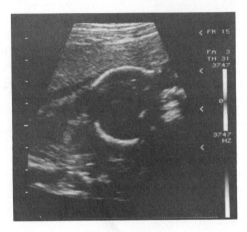

Figure 5-18. Fetal sonogram at approximately 20 weeks' gestation. (Courtesy of Benita Barthel, Ochsner Medical Foundation, New Orleans, Louisiana.)

This is the study of a 23-year-old gravida 1, para 0 female at approximately 20 weeks' gestation, who was referred to our department because of suspicion of a cranial abnormality seen on ultrasound at another institution. Other diagnostic studies revealed an elevated afAFP amniotic fluid, and 46XY normal male karyotype.

224. Sonographic findings in Figure 5-18 are highly suggestive of:
  A. hydrocephalus.
  B. holoprosencephaly.
  C. cystic hygroma.
  D. encephalocele.

225. The most common location for the occurrence of this abnormality is the:
  A. cisterna magna.
  B. occipital bone.
  C. parietal bone.
  D. fourth ventricle.

226. Other sonographically visible abnormalities that may be associated with this condition include:
  A. syndactyly and polycystic kidneys.
  B. polydactyly and multicystic kidneys.
  C. polydactyly and renal agenesis.
  D. syndactyly and renal agenesis.

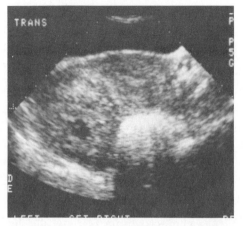

A

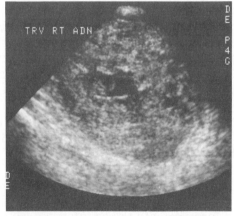

B

Figure 5-19. (*A*) Transabdominal pelvic scan. (*B*) Transvaginal adnexal scan. (Courtesy of Adele Hoffman and Kathy Dopson, Glengary, West Virginia.)

A 27-year-old female with a past history of ectopic pregnancy presented with complaints of amenorrhea and dull, right-sided pelvic pain. The patient is referred to rule out ectopic pregnancy. Transabdominal and transvaginal scans (Fig. 5-19) revealed the presence of a normal uterus demonstrating endometrial thickening but no evidence of an intrauterine pregnancy. In the right adnexa is a 5 cm × 8 cm complex mass, surrounding an intact gestational sac containing what appears to be embryonic or fetal echoes.

227. Based on the images presented, what is the location of the ectopic pregnancy?
    A. Within the interstitial portion of the tube
    B. In the cornual portion of the uterus
    C. Within the ampullary portion of the tube
    D. On the ovary

ANSWERS

1. B. The subdivisions of intrauterine life are the period of the ovum (the first 2 weeks), the period of the embryo (from the 3rd through the 8th week), and the period of the fetus.[8]

2. B. The ovaries of postmenopausal women are usually small (2 × 2 × 1 cm) and featureless, whereas the normal ovaries of a premenopausal woman can range up to 5 × 3 × 2 cm.[25] Ovarian atrophy generally occurs between 3 to 5 years after menopause. Depletion of the primordial egg cells and a relative lack of estrogen manifest in total cessation of menstrual function.[31]

3. B. For clinical purposes, macrosomia is generally defined as a fetal weight in excess of 4000 g, or a birth weight above the 90th percentile for gestational age. There are two main forms of macrosomia: symmetric and asymmetric. Symmetric or "constitutional" macrosomia is more commonly noted in patients with large stature and tends to recur in subsequent pregnancies. Asymmetric macrosomia occurs in diabetic patients where head and femur measurements vary in size and length but fall below the 90th percentile. Fetal abdominal circumference is particularly sensitive to insulin levels and so liver size can be monitored. When both abdominal circumference and fetal weight exceed the 90th percentile, the diagnosis of macrosomia is made.[5,56]

4. D. The two umbilical arteries, which carry most of the fetal aortic blood to the placenta, can be followed caudally from the anterior abdominal wall cord insertion site to the internal iliac arteries, just lateral to the bladder.[5] (Courtesy of Dayna Landru and Tracy Pfizenmaier, St. Francis Hospital School of Diagnostic Medical Sonography, Milwaukee, Wisconsin.)

5. A. Fertilization normally occurs in the distal third of the fallopian tube.[5,57,67]

6. C. The umbilical cord usually contains two arteries and one vein surrounded by mucoid connective tissue, often called Wharton's jelly.[32,43]

7. D. Alobar holoprosencephaly results in the replacement of the two lateral cerebral ventricles with a single midline ventricle and fusion of the thalami.[5,33,43]

8. B. The mature ovum or sperm each have 23 chromosomes. The

union of the ovum and sperm results in a cell with the full complement of 46 chromosomes (23 pairs), half contributed by the mother and half by the father.[8]

9. D. Sonographic documentation of an adnexal mass or pelvic intraperitoneal fluid in a woman with measurable circulation hCG and no evidence of an intrauterine pregnancy substantially increases her risk of harboring an extrauterine gestation.[12,65] (Courtesy of Lisa Elbert, Community College of Allegheny County, Monroeville, Pennsylvania.)

10. B. The Krukenberg tumor is a pathologic entity that describes ovarian metastases. Almost all tumors in this category have metastasized from the gastrointestinal tract, particularly from the colon.[26]

11. D. Morphologically, a corpus luteum is a thick-walled, noncystic structure that may attain a size up to 2 cm. From a practical pathologic perspective, the corpus luteum is called "cystic" when it exceeds 3 cm. It is the central zone that organizes into a cyst; the gelatinous liquid contained therein is fibrin.[12,31]

12. 1. E, 2. D, 3. G, 4. H, 5. A, 6. B, 7. C, 8. F[45]

13. C. Ovarian cysts in prepubescent or early pubescent females have been associated with juvenile hypothyroidism. In such cases, when drug therapy is successful in alleviating the thyroid malfunction, it is common to see resolution of the ovarian cysts.[42]

14. B. As a rule the uterus lies behind the bladder and is usually slightly tilted anteriorly (antiflexed). However, the uterus may be retroverted (pointing backward) as a normal variant.[17,57,61] (Courtesy of Amy Stillman, Orange Coast College, Costa Mesa, California.)

15. B. The estimation of serum levels of hCG is clinically superior to the measurement of any other pregnancy protein or biochemical parameter. With intrauterine pregnancy, hCG normally becomes detectable in the bloodstream 7 to 10 days after ovulation.[5,53]

16. C. To determine renal enlargement *in utero*, the ratio of the kidney circumference (in cross-section) to the abdominal circumference should not exceed 33%.[5,12,24,57]

17. B. In most tubal pregnancies, pain and subsequent tubal rupture occur at approximately 6 to 8 weeks' gestation.[64]

18. C. The gonads are derived from three sources: the coelomic epithelium, the underlying mesenchyme, and the primordial germ cells.[43] (Courtesy of Linda Foreman, Orange Coast College, Costa Mesa, California.)

19. C. The endometrium is approximately 5 to 7 mm in the secretory phase. In postmenopausal patients in the absence of estrogen replacement treatment, the endometrium, when visualized, is approximately 1 to 3 mm. An endometrial echo greater than 5 mm in such patients should be considered abnormal and investigated further.[12, 28]

20. 1. E, 2. F, 3. C, 4. A, 5. D, 6. B[45]

21. C. The fetal heart rate is usually 120 to 160 beats per minute and is thus easily distinguished from the maternal pulse.[37, 46]

22. B. Diethylstilbestrol (DES)-exposed females are at increased risk of pregnancy complications such as ectopic pregnancy, first-trimester abortion, and premature labor. Premature labor may be caused in part by an incompetent cervix, another side effect of DES exposure.[5, 54, 61] (Courtesy of Linda Foreman, Orange Coast College, Costa Mesa, California.)

23. C. One of the late-developing fetal systems is the fetal urinary system. Kidneys are usually developed *in utero* by a gestational age of 15 weeks.[5, 12, 43, 53]

24. B. A meningocele is a spinal defect associated with spina bifida, which causes the meninges to project through the defect in the vertebral arches. A cystic swelling is formed beneath the skin and contains cerebrospinal fluid which communicates with the subarachnoid space. The spinal cord and nerves are usually normal.[67] (Courtesy of Bonnie Kazor, Community College of Allegheny County, Monroeville, Pennsylvania.)

25. C. Quantifiable levels of hCG are present by 10 days following ovulation. The doubling time for beta-hCG in normal gestations ranges from 1.2 to 3.2 days, with a mean of 2.2 days.[56] (Courtesy of Janie Hay, Orange Coast College, Costa Mesa, California.)

26. C. An easily performed and sensitive measurement for the exclusion of ventriculomegaly is the sonographic measurement of the atrium of the lateral ventricle at the region of the glomus of the choroid plexus.[34]

27. A. The cause of leiomyomas (fibroids) is unknown. It appears that leiomyoma development may be related to estrogen stimulation. This is supported by the fact that myomas are not commonly seen before menarche and usually do not grow after menopause. It is also reported that myomas grow rapidly in situations in which there is unopposed estrogen activity. Fibroids sometimes enlarge during pregnancy because of pregnancy-related estrogen levels.[5, 47, 53]

28. C. In coexisting pregnancy and a mass, it is important during follow-up examinations to make precise measurements since the mass may have changed position and location, and also because some masses—like the cystadenoma—tend to grow during pregnancy.[5, 56] (Courtesy of Stephanie Ellingson, University of Iowa Hospitals and Clinics, Iowa City, Iowa.)

29. A. Amniotic sheets are commonly occurring structures that appear to be composed of 2 layers of apposed *amniochorionic membrane*, resulting in 4 distinct histologic layers. They closely resemble the "thick" diamniotic-dichorionic membranes associated with twins.[22, 68]

30. D. Duodenal obstruction usually results in a classic "double bubble" appearance of the stomach and duodenal bulb.[1, 48] (Courtesy of Gail Gould, Orange Coast College, Costa Mesa, California.)

31. D. Transperineal scanning has specific indications from mid-trimester to term pregnancies and at the beginning of labor, which transabdominal and transvaginal scanning cannot meet or can only partially fulfill. These include cervical evaluation in late third trimester to term pregnancies; diagnosis of PROM (premature rupture of the membranes); establishment of the placental relationship with the internal cervical os; diagnosis of cervical effacement and dilatation in early labor; and the imaging of fetal anatomy.[16, 70]

32. E

33. B

34. J

35. C

36. H

37. F

38. A

39. I

40. G

41. D[45]

42. C. In a normal ovulatory cycle, one follicle becomes dominant and ruptures through the tunica albuginea, releasing its contained egg. The typical mature follicle reaches 20 mm in size before rupturing.[5, 56]

43. B. An abnormally low msAFP is used to screen fetuses at risk of having chromosomal trisomy. Down's syndrome (trisomy 21) is sometimes associated with a decreased level of msAFP.[5, 12, 66] (Courtesy of Jennifer Cooper-Wilson, Orange Coast College, Costa Mesa, California.)

44. B. In a study of the endometrial thickness in postmenopausal women, Granberg et al. established 5 mm as the normal limit.[28]

45. C. Dermoid cysts may contain a significant amount of hair. In fact, the fat and hair within them can contribute to their appearance as an echogenic mass. This situation has been termed the *tip of the iceberg* sign, indicating that only the most proximal portion of the echogram mass will be delineated.[54, 56] (Courtesy of Benita Barthel, Ochsner Medical Foundation, New Orleans, Louisiana.)

46. D. Interstitial pregnancy occurs with implantation in the interstitial segment of the fallopian tube traversing the uterine wall. Because of the relationship of the interstitial tubal segment to the uterine wall, it is possible to sonographically demonstrate a myometrial mantle in intact interstitial pregnancies. When rupture does occur, patients are at great risk of exsanguination because of the abundant blood supply to the region by both the ovarian and uterine arteries. Precise early diagnosis permits conservative non-surgical treatment with methotrexate.[62]

47. D. Today, using high-frequency transvaginal probes, the discriminatory hCG zone is in the range of 1025 IU/ml (IRP) or 300 to 750 mIU/ml (2nd I.S.).[5] (Courtesy of Laura Hodge, Orange Coast College, Costa Mesa, California.)

48. C. The first structure to be visualized sonographically within the gestational sac is the secondary yolk sac.[5, 12]

49. B. Several sonographic features aid in the diagnosis of cystic hygroma. First, the septi dividing the dilated lymphatic channels are usually quite thick and exceed the width of cyst walls noted with branchial cysts, meningoceles, or encephaloceles. Second, non-immune hydrops often develops secondary to lymphatic obstruction.[12,56] (Courtesy of Michelle Bolitho, Orange Coast College, Costa Mesa, California.)

50. D. The risk of Down's syndrome is increased when the ratio of femur and humerus to BPD is 0.9 or less. A thickened nuchal fold (6 mm or greater) is the most reliable sign between 14 to 20 weeks' gestation. Approximately 25% of affected fetuses will demonstrate decreased AFP levels.[13,29]

51. C. Occasionally, a normal-looking gestational sac may be partially surrounded by a crescent-shaped sonolucent collection. This is evidence of a subchorionic hemorrhage (bleeding between the endometrium and the gestational sac). Coexistence of a subchorionic hemorrhage with embryonic heart activity leads to a slightly reduced continuation rate (30% fail to continue to term).[5]

52. A. Fetal heart rates of approximately 80 to 85 beats per minute can normally be detected with transvaginal scanning during the late 4th or early 5th menstrual week.[20]

53. C. Sonographically visible lower extremity epiphyseal ossification centers in the distal femur and proximal tibia can be useful in the evaluation of fetal age and lung maturity. The presence of ossification sites in the distal femoral epiphyses indicates a menstrual age of at least 33 weeks.[12] (Courtesy of Jo Addington, Orange Coast College, Costa Mesa, California.)

54. B. Initially, alfa fetoprotein is produced in the embryologic yolk sac and later by the fetal liver. At any time during gestation, levels of AFP in the fetal serum are 100 to 10,000 times greater than those found in maternal serum, with the highest gradients occurring in earlier gestation. Therefore, elevation of msAFP levels can occur whenever small amounts of fetal blood enter the maternal circulation.[10,66]

55. D. The criterion for accurate measurement of the nuchal fold is measurement from the outer limit of the occipital bone to the skin edge, using a modified transverse view of the fetal head that includes the brain stem, cerebellum, and occipital bone. A nuchal fold of 6 mm or more is considered a positive indicator of abnormality.[3]

56. C. Fertilization occurs with contact of a spermatozoon with an ovum followed by fusion. This stimulates and completes ovum maturation, which leads to the formation of a zygote.[12, 67]

57. B. A coexisting complete mole and a normal fetus in a normal gestational sac arise from transformation of the trophoblast of one of the two dizygotic twin placentas. The findings should be confirmed histologically, as these lesions are considered to have the same malignant potential as the more classic hydatidiform mole.[5, 12, 57]

58. C. Klinefelter syndrome is a condition involving the male reproductive tract and is unrelated to omphalocele. Omphaloceles are associated with trisomies 13, 15, 16, and, to a lesser extent, with trisomy 21.[12, 43] (Courtesy of Carrie Robbins, Orange Coast College, Costa Mesa, California.)

59. B. In a study by Goldstein and Snyder evaluating the significance of embryonic cardiac activity, it was determined that the absence of cardiac activity in embryos 4 mm or greater was reliably associated with embryonic demise.[26, 27]

60. B. The fetal bladder normally fills and empties every 15 to 45 minutes; therefore, it is necessary to extend the examination of any fetus (from 15 weeks on) in which the bladder is not visualized.[50]

61. D. A vein of Galen abnormality represents an arteriovenous malformation which appears as an oval or tubular cystic area just above and behind the thalamus. The defect usually does not exceed 2.5 cm in its smallest diameter, and is often accompanied by heterogeneous cystic areas around the larger lucent aneurysm, which represent dilated blood vessels.[15]

62. A. The rare condition of twin embolization syndrome may occur after one of the twins sharing the placenta dies *in utero*. Infarcts in the surviving twin can cause structural and functional changes, presumably due to embolization of debris, thrombus, thromboplastic material, and toxins from the dying twin's circulation. The surviving twin is at risk of developing brain defects, intestinal atresia, renal dysplasia or necrosis, extremity abnormalities, and cutaneous skin defects.[30, 52]

63. A. When evaluating the fetal heart it is necessary to use not only the standard four-chamber view, but also outflow-tract views, to avoid missing such defects as transposition of the great arteries and tetralogy of Fallot.[7]

64. C. If the diagnosis can be established early, cervical cerclage may save the pregnancy in a woman with an incompetent cervix.[12] (Courtesy of Jo Addington, Orange Coast College, Costa Mesa, California.)

65. C. The finger-like fimbriae of the uterine tube move back and forth over the ovary at ovulation, "sweeping" the ovum into the infundibulum of the tube.[43]

66. B. Female offspring exposed to diethylstilbestrol (DES) during pregnancy may have a variety of uterine abnormalities that can be detected sonographically. Among them are the T-shaped uterus, which has been described as a uterus lacking the normal bulbous nature of the uterine fundus. Care must be taken to assure that the full AP diameter of the uterine fundus is shown on sagittal scans before this diagnosis is chosen.[56]

67. C. Meckel's syndrome (or Meckel-Gruber syndrome) was first described by Meckel in 1822 and subsequently by Gruber in 1934. It is an autosomal recessive disorder with many associated deformities. Major features include multicystic dysplastic kidneys, occipital encephalocele, and postaxial polydactyly. Two of these three major features are sufficient to make the diagnosis.[60]

68. B. The proper technique for measuring the femur is to select the femur closest to the transducer, measure the diaphyses (making sure the transducer is perpendicular to the bone shaft), and correlate the femur measurements with measurements of the BPD and abdomen circumference.[5, 12, 41, 57] (Courtesy of Sheila Lind, Orange Coast College, Costa Mesa, California.)

69. B. In the midline, fibers from the levator ani insert on the walls of the rectum, vagina, and urethra as they pass through the pelvic diaphragm.[5, 67]

70. C. While carcinoma of the ovary is the third most common site of malignancy, it is the number one cause of death in women with cancer of the genital tract. Cervical carcinoma and endometrial carcinoma are first and second in frequency but second and third in terms of mortality. While deaths from cervical cancer are on the decline, deaths resulting from undetected endometrial cancers are on the rise.[51] (Courtesy of Amy Stillman, Orange Coast College, Costa Mesa, California.)

71. 1. D, 2. F, 3. A, 4. B, 5. C, 6. E[45]

72. C. The number and arrangement of internal septae within predominantly cystic masses do not appear to correlate with benign or malignant characteristics. However, the more solid or irregular areas within such a mass or on its surface, the more likely the possibility of malignancy.[56] (Courtesy of Michelle Guillory, Ochsner Medical Foundation, New Orleans, Louisiana.)

73. C. The walls of the uterus are composed of three tissue layers. The outermost layer consists of fascia that is continuous with the pelvic fascia and forms a *serous* covering that invests the uterine walls. The thick middle layer is composed of smooth muscle cells interspersed with connective tissue fibers. The endometrium is a *mucous* layer that varies in thickness and composition throughout the menstrual cycle.[5,6,7]

74. C. Because uterine anomalies occur in at least 50% of patients with developmental urinary tract disorders, such as renal agenesis and ectopic kidney, sonographers should make it a practice to examine both systems whenever an anomaly exists in either one.[5,12] (Courtesy of Susan Ley, Community College of Allegheny County, Monroeville, Pennsylvania.)

75. B. FSH, the follicle stimulating hormone, causes maturation of the ovarian follicle, and as a consequence, produces estrogen. Increased blood levels of estrogen inhibit the production of FSH and stimulate production of LH, the luteinizing hormone. A predominantly LH mixture causes ovulation. LH is responsible for the formation of the corpus luteum and the secretion of progesterone.[8]

76. C. The blastocyst stage follows the morula stage, when development of intercellular fluid increases and an inner cell mass is attached at one pole of the morula to the inner surface of the cells of the outer cell mass. The cells of the outer cell mass become flattened and are known as the *trophoblast*. The young embryo floats freely in the uterine cavity and is now ready to become attached to the uterine wall.[67] (Courtesy of Laura McNaughton, Orange Coast College, Costa Mesa, California.)

77. A. Previous curettage and, to a lesser extent, prior cesarean section, appear to be predisposing factors for the occurrence of synechiae, which may lead to the development of amniotic sheets in subsequent pregnancies.[21]

78. B. The most common site for implantation of ectopic pregnancies is the ampullary portion of the fallopian tube. The second most common site is the isthmus.[12,51,65]

79. B. Monochorionic twins result from the fertilization of a single egg by a single sperm and the "splitting" of the resulting products of conception into two identical parts. Because they share the exact same genetic heritage, the embryos will be of the same sex, blood type, and predisposition to disease.[5, 12, 46]

80. D. Initially the kidneys lie in the pelvis, but they migrate into the abdomen mainly from growth of the embryo's body caudal to the kidneys. As the kidneys move out of the pelvis they are supplied by arteries at successively higher levels. The caudal arteries normally degenerate as the kidney ascends and new vessels form. The majority of ectopic kidneys are located (but some are low) in the abdomen. Ectopic kidneys receive their blood supply from blood vessels near them and are often supplied by multiple vessels.[43] (Courtesy of Nancy Wityk, Johns Hopkins School of Diagnostic Medical Sonography, Baltimore, Maryland.)

81. D. Although the gallbladder volume increases during pregnancy, the upper limit of normal for bile duct diameter is 5 mm, which is the same as the general population. Therefore, the common duct size during pregnancy is unchanged.[59]

82. B. Neovascular vessels within malignant tumors lack a normal vessel's muscular coating. They are sinusoid-like and have numerous arteriovenous shunts. All of these factors contribute to the increased diastolic flow that is apparent on Doppler waveforms as low pulsatility.[25]

83. A. LGA fetuses face elevated risk for obstetrical complications during delivery. These include birth trauma, shoulder dystocia, meconium aspiration, and prolonged labor.[4]

84. D. Autopsy reports have demonstrated that the most common renal anomalies found in trisomy 13 infants are hyperlobulation, dysplasia, and the presence of cortical cysts.[5, 11, 12, 43]

85. A. The use of Doppler ultrasound in studying fetal blood flow has become commonplace. The greatest clinical application appears to be in IUGR, twin gestation, and, to a lesser extent, in postterm pregnancy and pregnancies complicated by systemic lupus erythematosus.[36, 52, 69]

86. A. Gartner's duct cysts develop from cystic dilatation of remnants of the embryonic mesonephrose. They are most commonly unilateral, single, and found in the anterolateral wall of the vagina. A Gartner's duct cyst shares similar sonographic patterns with other

vaginal abnormalities, such as abscesses, hematomas, necrotic neoplasms, or even endometriosis.[49]

87. 1. B, 2. H, 3. M, 4. E, 5. K, 6. D, 7. N, 8. I, 9. A, 10. L, 11. J, 12. F, 13. G, 14. C[45]

88. D. Most sonographic reports of talipes equinovarus are characterized sonographically by constant visualization of the long axis of the foot on the same plane of section, but at right angles to the tibia and fibula.[12,47,53]

89. B. The inner cell mass, or embryonic pole, differentiates into two layers: an outer layer of endoderm and an inner layer of ectoderm lying adjacent to the trophoblast. Within the ectoderm the amniotic cavity begins as a small fluid collection. Another fluid-filled structure forms adjacent to the endoderm. This cavity is the primitive yolk sac.[5,43]

90. D. Erythroblastosis fetalis is hemolytic anemia of the fetus caused by the transplacental passage of maternal antibodies, and is associated with severe Rh isoimmunization in pregnancy. Cleft lip or palate defect can be associated with a number of syndromes, with holoprosencephaly, other facial defects, and chromosomal aberrations including trisomy 13 and 18 and triploidy.[11,56]

91. B. Movement of the flap of the foramen ovale occurs within the left atrium, on the same side of the interatrial and interventricular septa as the left ventricle.[56]

92. A. Viral infections, such as cytomegalovirus and varicella zoster (chickenpox), produce a great number of associated fetal cerebral calcifications.[5,33]

93. C. The majority of ovarian follicles in patients taking birth control pills will be small, irregular, and atretic.[12]

94. B. Persistent truncus arteriosus results when the upper part of the bulbus cordis (the truncus arteriosus) does not become divided into the aorta and pulmonary trunk because of failure of the spiral aorticopulmonary septum to develop. In this condition, only one artery arises from the heart, and the pulmonary arteries originate from this single trunk.[67]

95. D. Sarcoma botryoides is the most common malignant vaginal and uterine lesion of young girls. Symptoms include bloody vaginal dis-

charge. Primary adenocarcinoma of the uterus has been reported in daughters of mothers exposed to diethylstilbestrol (DES). It presents with vaginal bleeding and a rapidly growing tumor not associated with sexual precocity. The discovery of foreign objects within the vagina is increasing with the rise in the incidence of sexual child abuse.[5]

96. D. Reverberation and multipath artifacts can be corrected by using transducers of a different frequency or scanning the same area from a different angle. In the case of bladder artifacts it is additionally helpful to reduce the volume of urine in the bladder before rescanning.[5,57]

97. A. Gammete intrafallopian transfer (GIFT) is an alternative to *in vitro* fertilization–embryo transfer in patients with demonstrated tubal patency of at least one tube. Sperm and ovum are deposited by a catheter (inserted into the aspirating needle of a laparoscope) in the ampullary region of the fallopian tube.[5]

98. D. Spina bifida refers to a defect in the spine resulting from a failure of the two halves of the vertebral arch to fuse. These lesions usually occur in the lumbosacral and cervical regions. If the meninges protrudes through the defect (spina bifida cystica), the lesion is designated a meningocele; if neural tissue is included, it is called a meningomyelocele. With spina bifida occulta there is a bony defect without protrusion of cord or meninges.[5,12,43] (Courtesy of Ed Marsh, Orange Coast College, Costa Mesa, California.)

99. C. The fetal aorta serves as a constant sonolucent landmark as it courses through the fetal abdomen. In the physiologically sound fetus, the fluid-filled stomach and urine-filled bladder serve as dynamically changing but highly visible anatomical landmarks.[5,57]

100. C. Normal corpus luteum cysts are expected to regress after 14 to 15 weeks' gestation.[5,12]

101. C. L/S stands for lecithin/sphingomyelin. From the 24th menstrual week of gestation the alveolar phase of lung development generally begins and extends into postnatal life. During this period the alveolar cells secrete phospholipids (surfactant) that play a key role in the functional integrity of the fetal lung at delivery. If these phospholipids are not present in sufficient quantities at birth, the fetal alveoli will collapse, and the fetus will receive inadequate oxygenation. Such fetuses are at risk for respiratory distress syndrome or hyaline membrane disease. This condition usually affects fetuses that are born prematurely.[12]

102. B. Patients who are referred for study of the umbilical artery wave-forms should have completed all prior testing. Maternal position-ing should remain constant throughout the test, with the patient placed in the semi-recumbent position with left lateral tilt, prior to obtaining the umbilical artery waveforms.[69]

103. D. The echoes of structures distal to a cyst demonstrate increased echo amplitudes, beginning at the far wall and proceeding distally. This increased amplitude is better known as the *acoustic enhance-ment artifact*. It occurs because tissue located on either side of the cystic structure attenuate more sound than does the cystic structure.[5]

104. C. At C-section delivery, the sonographic diagnosis of sacral coc-cygeal teratoma was confirmed. The fetus survived and was report-edly doing well.[33, 47]

105. C. The space of Retzius, also known as the prevesical or retropubic space, is situated between the transversalis fascia and the umbilical prevesical fascia. Sonographically, masses in the space of Retzius are usually hematomas or abscesses, and are capable of displacing the bladder posteriorly if they achieve a large size.[12]

106. C. A new, easier method of sonographically detecting cleft lips is to observe the closed lips to avoid false positive findings that may be created by imaging the normal frenulum of the upper lip.[33, 47, 53, 63]

107. D. The placental lucency most likely represents a venous lake; how-ever, a small chorioangioma cannot be ruled out.

108. D. Toxemia of pregnancy is a disease occurring in the third trimes-ter. Characterized by maternal edema, hypertension, proteinuria, and central nervous system irritability, the disease has been classi-fied into two stages, preeclampsia and eclampsia. The preeclamptic stage is marked by development of hypertension with proteinuria or edema, or both. In the eclamptic stage, one or more convulsions will occur, significantly increasing the risk of maternal and fetal mortality.[5]

109. B. Only 10% to 20% of pregnancies attain a grade III placenta by term.[5, 12]

110. D. Gastroschisis is an abdominal wall defect usually located 2 to 4 cm from the midline (typically to the right), and unrelated to the umbilical cord. The herniated viscera are not covered by any mem-brane or sac. Sonographic diagnosis is assured by the presence of free-floating, small bowel loops in the amniotic fluid.[5, 33, 47, 53]

111. B. An accumulation of serous fluid in the subcutaneous connective tissue and the serous cavities of the body is an ominous sign and can be collectively referred to as *anasarca*.[45]

112. D. Normal mild dilatation of the fetal renal collecting system ranges between 3 to 11 mm.[6, 11]

113. A. Chorioangioma represents one of the two primary, nontrophoblastic tumors of the placenta. It is a vascular malformation that occurs on the fetal surface of the placenta, often adjacent to the cord insertion. Large chorioangiomas may cause significant vascular shunting. Compression of the cord vessels by an expanding tumor can cause "fetal asphyxiation."[5, 47, 56]

114. D. Clinically significant retained placenta tissue is unlikely when ultrasound demonstrates a normally appearing uterine stripe, isolated endometrial fluid, or hyperechoic foci without an associated mass. Echogenic foci seen in the uterus after instrumentation are frequently caused by air rather than retained placenta. Therefore, whenever possible ultrasound should be performed before instrumentation in patients with suspected retained products of conception (RPC).[35]

115. D. Abruption may manifest itself in three ways: as external bleeding without significant intrauterine hematoma, as formation of a retroplacental or marginal hematoma, and as formation of a submembranous clot at a distance from the placenta. The sonographic appearance varies depending on location and age of the hemorrhage. Differential diagnosis must include hydatidiform mole, chorioangioma, and normal but engorged myometrial veins in the subplacental complex.[5]

116. B. The ultrasound diagnosis was uterine fibroids causing retroversion of the uterus. The density of fibroids is a known factor in posterior bladder wall displacements and decreased posterior sound transmission.[12, 57]

117. C. Toxemia of pregnancy is a disease that occurs in the third trimester. The condition is characterized by maternal edema, hypertension, proteinuria, and central nervous system irritability.[5]

118. C. Adenomyosis is endometriosis of the myometrium. In three-quarters of cases there is uterine enlargement. Small hypoechoic areas, resulting from hemorrhage or secretions, are sometimes found within the area of invasion.[56]

119. B. The cisterna magna is seen in scans taken at the cerebellar level, and can be measured between the vermis and the inner table of the occipital bone.[5]

120. B. A sydrome is a group of symptoms and signs, which, when considered together, characterize a disease or lesion.[5,47]

121. A. The most frequent cause of congenital hydrocephaly is aqueductal stenosis, which is suggested by the symmetric or asymmetric enlargement of the lateral and third ventricles in the presence of the fourth ventricle. Aqueductal stenosis is caused by obstruction or narrowing of the aqueduct of Sylvius.[47]

122. B. Omphaloceles may contain bowel and liver. Those containing bowel alone are associated with an underlying chromosomal disorder.[47,53]

123. C. A full urinary bladder is essential to elevate and reposition the uterus for transabdominal scanning in a nongravid patient. Time permitting, rehydrating the patient and waiting a sufficient amount of time for the bladder to begin filling would be the first choice in this situation.[16,41]

124. D. When fetal position prevents adequate demonstration of the lower uterine segment, especially in a case of placenta previa, the sonographer may try a variety of maneuvers to achieve adequate visualization of the placenta. Before the fetal head descends below the level of the sacral promontory, placing the patient in trendelenburg position may produce a favorable change in fetal position. If this maneuver is unsuccessful, the sonographer should measure the distance between the fetal skull and the sacral promontory. A distance greater than 1.5 cm indicates that a previa cannot be ruled out. Supplemental translabial or transperineal scans will demonstrate the presence of placental tissue covering the internal cervical os.[16,41]

125. D. Sonography can frequently distinguish abnormal from normal "empty" gestational sacs on a single examination, independent of menstrual history. An anembryonic pregnancy is one that demonstrates absence of an embryo in a gestational sac greater than 25 mm, or a gestational sac greater than 20 mm that lacks a yolk sac.[5,12]

126. C. One of the characteristic signs of the Arnold-Chiari malformation is the lemon sign. The lemon sign describes an indentation or scal-

loping of the frontal bones. This finding should alert the sonographer to search for an unsuspected spina bifida.[5, 33]

127. B. As a general rule, after 23 weeks the placenta should be no thinner than 1.5 cm or thicker than 5.0 cm.[5, 19, 56]

128. D. The chorion and amnion have distinct embryologic origins and exist as separate membranes until about the 16th week. Progressive fusion of the chorion to the amnion begins in mid–first trimester and progresses until the 16th week with obliteration of the chorionic cavity.[5, 12]

129. D. Intrauterine growth retardation is usually defined as birthweight less than the 10th percentile for gestational age. Intrinsic or symmetric types arise from conditions within the fetal compartment itself: chromosomal abnormalities, early intrauterine infections, embryonic teratogenic insults and genetic factors. Extrinsic or asymmetric IUGR results from nutrient limitation.[44]

130. C

131. D

132. B

133. A

134. F[5, 43]

135. B. Sebum within a cystic teratoma may collect anteriorly, presenting a fat-fluid layer pattern.[25]

136. A. At approximately 7 weeks' gestational age, the rhombencephalon will appear as a prominent hypoechoic area within the posterior aspect of the brain.[5, 57]

137. B. Longitudinal cervical length measurements vary from 2.5 to 5.0 cm in healthy pregnancies. In cases of incompetent cervix the measurements are 2.0 to 4.0 cm.[25]

138. D. The uterus widens toward the fundus and the cornual regions, the lateral triangular areas extending bilaterally from the fundus. It is the cornu that are the points of origin for the fallopian tubes.[5, 8, 43, 57]

139. D. In approximately 10% of monochorionic pregnancies there is no separating membrane indicating the presence of a monoamniotic pregnancy. Absence of a separating membrane suggests the possibility of many associated anomalies, including conjoined twins, locking twins, polyhydramnios, and asymmetrical growth.[57]

140. B. Polyhydramnios is associated with diabetic pregnancy, multiple pregnancy, hydrops, and viral infections. However, a normal variant—idiopathic hydramnios—may occur. Most frequently, idiopathic hydramnios takes place between 20 to 30 weeks' gestation.[57]

141. B. The appearance of hirsutism, oligomenorrhea, and infertility, as well as bilaterally enlarged ovaries containing multiple 1- to 2-mm size cysts describe the Stein-Leventhal syndrome.[57]

142. D. A low head-to-abdomen ratio suggests the possibility of microcephalus or a large fetus with macrosomia.[57]

143. D. Three possibilities should be considered whenever a fetus is suspiciously small for dates: the mother's dates are wrong and the fetus is actually younger than indicated by her dates; palpation is misleading because of obesity or unusual uterine lie; and oligohydramnios is present owing to premature rupture of the membranes, IUGR, or fetal renal anomalies.[56,57]

144. B. First trimester crown-rump length measurement is the optimal method of establishing fetal age. Correct measurement requires finding the longest axis of the fetus. This measurement can be readily obtained from approximately 7 to 12 weeks (LMP). The crown-rump length measurements are inaccurate after 12 weeks' gestation.[5,12,18,41,57]

145. C. The most practical and efficacious method of disinfection is to spray the probe with a disinfectant before use. Sporicidin is sufficiently bacteriostatic and virostatic (including the HIV virus) since it kills on contact. Cidex is another recommended preparation which may require immersion in the solution for a specified period of time. Some manufacturers, but not all, recommend the use of 1 part bleach per 10 parts water or gas sterilization. Selection of appropriate disinfectants should follow manufacturers' recommendations and directions to prevent voiding the transducer warranty.[25]

146. D. Ovarian fibromas are the tumor most often associated with Meigs' syndrome. The characteristics of this syndrome include pel-

)   /

vic mass, hydrothorax, and ascites with right chest pleural effusion most common. The unique trait of Meigs' syndrome is that the characteristics resolve after tumor removal.[12, 40]

147. D. With acute PID, sonography typically demonstrates adnexal or cul-de-sac fluid collections that are irregularly shaped and echogenic. There may also be increased echogenicity of the endometrial canal including separation due to fluid build-up. Irregular, thick-walled cul-de-sac and cystic to complex masses located lateral, posterior, or superior to the uterus may also occur. Additionally, fluid-fluid levels may also develop, and most likely represent pyosalpinx or tubo-ovarian abscesses. Tissue edema produces a loss of interfaces and blurring of the margins between pelvic structures, as well.[5, 12, 57]

148. C. When a pregnant patient lies in the supine position, a large gravid uterus may cause compression of the inferior vena cava and possibly lower the blood pressure, causing her to feel faint and possibly nauseated. This condition is known as *supine hypotension syndrome*. A change in patient position from supine to left lateral decubitus alleviates the problem in the shortest period of time, as it rapidly relieves the pressure on the vena cava.[12, 39, 41]

149. B. When the sound beam is perpendicular to an IUD, an acoustic shadow is demonstrated if the IUD falls within the narrow portion of the beam. To narrow the beam, a high-frequency or focused transducer is used. The gain is usually adjusted to a lower setting to prevent noise from obscuring the image.[5]

150. D. Common sites of metastases from pelvic malignancies are the retroperitoneal nodes, peritoneal surfaces, omentum, and in some specific malignancies, the liver.[12, 33]

151. D. Pseudocyesis is defined as "false pregnancy." The patient develops all the signs of a pregnancy without the presence of any intrauterine products of conception or a positive pregnancy test.[5, 9]

152. D. The coding system used to document a patient's reproductive history usually follows this method: *Gravidity* (G) refers to the number of pregnancies the patient has had and includes the current one. As an example, a pregnant woman who had an ectopic pregnancy and gave birth to twins would be G3. *Parity* (P) refers to the number of pregnancies the patient has carried to term; thus, an ectopic pregnancy would be recorded as P1 and a twin gestation would be P1. The numbers used after P refer, in the order pre-

Brachy – short
Dolico – long

sented, to the number of term pregnancies, premature deliveries, abortions, and living children. Thus, G4P1012 indicates that the patient has been pregnant 4 times (including the current pregnancy), has had 1 full-term pregnancy, no premature deliveries, 1 abortion (the ectopic pregnancy), and two full-term births, in this case, a set of twins.[5]

153. A. Variations in fetal head shape can significantly alter the accuracy of the BPD in predicting fetal age. The most commonly encountered head-shape variation is dolichocephaly, the presence of a flattened, elongated skull. Dolichocephaly is often seen in breech fetuses, twins, and cases of oligohydramnios. Brachycephaly may also be encountered in twin gestations and can be seen in some forms of dwarfism and Down's syndrome. In cases of unusual head shape, a head circumference measurement is usually more accurate than a BPD.[1,33]

154. C. As development proceeds, a large channel—the ductus venosus—develops in the liver and connects the umbilical vein with the inferior vena cava. The ductus venosus acts as a bypass through the liver, enabling some blood from the placenta to pass almost directly to the heart. After birth, the ductus venosus becomes obliterated and fibrosed and forms the *ligamentum venosum*, and the left umbilical vein forms a similar ligament in the free margin of the falciform ligament, called the *ligamentum teres*. This extends from the umbilicus to the porta hepatis of the liver.[43,67]

155. A. Arrhenoblastoma is the most common androgen-secreting tumor. It produces masculinization, amenorrhea, and infertility. Granulosa cell tumors are feminizing neoplasms composed of cells resembling the graffian follicle. They can produce precocious puberty in prepubertal victims, and endometrial hyperplasia and bleeding in postmenopausal patients.[56,57]

156. B. A gestational sac usually grows at a rate of 1 to 1.1 mm/day or 3.5 cm/wk.[25]

157. A. Tubo-ovarian abscesses (TOAs) are usually bilateral, but occasionally a unilateral lesion is seen. The TOAs are irregularly shaped, thick-walled, fluid-filled structures situated in the adnexa, and may develop a few internal echoes and even an internal fluid-fluid level.[56,57]

158. D. The exact etiology of abruptio placentae is not known; however, it has been observed that placental abruptions are much more com-

mon in women with high parity, increased maternal age, chronic hypertension, dietary folic acid deficiency, congenital uterine anomalies, and trauma (which would also include amniocentesis).[46]

159. C. The demonstration of a perisac sonolucent area between 6 and 8 weeks of pregnancy is a normal variant, thought to represent implantation bleeding.[12, 27, 56, 57]

160. B. Although there is a normal decline in the amount of amniotic fluid during the waning days of pregnancy, with postmaturity there is usually outright oligohydramnios. With Potter's syndrome, renal agenesis prevents production of urine and routinely leads to oligohydramnios. IUGR is associated with oligohydramnios, but duodenal atresia (like other swallowing defects) is most often associated with the production of polyhydramnios.[5, 12, 57]

161. A. In a frank breech presentation (most common), the thighs are flexed at the hips with the legs and knees extended. In complete breech (least common), the thighs are flexed at the hips, and there is flexion of the knees as well. One or both hips and knees are extended in the footling breech.[12, 46]

162. C. Since many fetal organs are not bilateral, several transverse sections will convey important information concerning the position of the fetus. Each time you measure a BPD, you demonstrate the thalamus. The thalami are heart-shaped, and the apex of this heart points toward the spine of the fetus. Therefore, in only one scan you can deduce the position of the head (vertex or breech) and the position of the spine (left or right).[33, 38, 53]

163. A. Early use of RhoGam was limited to administration following delivery of an Rh-positive fetus to an Rh-negative mother. To prevent sensitization in this setting, RhoGam must be administered within 72 hours (3 days) of delivery. Its use is now widely recommended for the management of nonsensitized Rh-negative gravidas after 20 weeks as a prophylactic measure.[2, 5, 12, 56]

164. B. Decidualized endometrium can be seen to have three distinct layers, defined by their relationship to the blastocyst. The decidua capsularis closes over and surrounds the blastocyst. The decidua parietalis, or decidua vera, is the decidua that lines the remainder of the endometrial cavity. The decidua basalis develops at the point of attachment by the blastocyst and will contribute the maternal portion of the placenta.[5, 12, 43]

165. B

166. A

167. B

168. A

169. D

170. B

171. A

172. A

173. C

174. A[5,43,46]

175. A. CAM Type II is typically a unilateral condition that leads to the development of pathologic mass consisting of multiple uniform-sized cysts of about 1 to 1.5 cm in diameter. There are associated renal, cardiac, and gastrointestinal malformations; as with all space-occupying lung masses, there may be associated fetal hydrops, ascites, and polyhydramnios.[5,33]

176. A. The accuracy of the predictive value of the BPD has been reported as ± 1 week at 16 weeks' gestation. Its accuracy diminishes with fetal age from approximately 32 to 33 weeks' gestation. Consequently, if the BPD is being used to estimate fetal age, the measurements should be performed before 33 weeks LMP.[5,41,57]

177. C. Factors that increase risk of ectopic pregnancy are prior ectopic pregnancy, pregnancy with IUD in place, history of pelvic inflammatory disease, prior tubal reconstructive surgery, fertility drug or oral contraceptive therapy, pregnancy by *in vitro* fertilization, and pregnancy after laparoscopic tubal coagulation.[55,65]

178. D. Sonographers' pretap responsibilities include documenting the location of a suitable pocket of fluid that is free of fetal parts, the umbilical cord, and if possible, the placenta. It is also important to document the location of the maternal bladder, and to recheck the selected tap site following patient voiding if the amniocentesis procedure will be carried out after any considerable time interval or without continuous ultrasound guidance.[5,12,56]

179. D. Not more than 15% to 20% of pregnancies attain a grade III placenta appearance by term. Basal and interlobar septal calcifications and other signs of the grade III placenta are expected from 38 weeks of gestation.[5, 12, 57]

180. C. Subserosal fibroids are frequently pedunculated and may simulate adnexal masses.[12, 33, 56]

181. D. Theca lutein cysts, though seen in normal pregnancy, are most commonly associated with multiple gestation, trophoblastic disease (30%), or ovarian hyperstimulation syndrome (20% to 40%), and a variety of conditions that result in fetal hydrops.[56]

182. B. CVS is performed between 8 and 12 weeks after the last menstrual period. Laboratory results are obtainable within 48 hours by short-term culture method. This is backed by long-term culture method, which provides results in 4 to 7 days.[5, 32]

183. C. Abdominal measurements have a much higher rate of intraobserver and interobserver variability than biparietal or femur length measurements. The first step is to obtain a section of the abdomen that is as round as possible, one that is devoid of rib, and one in which the *umbilical portion* of the left portal vein or bifurcation of the portal vein should lie directly opposite the fetal spine.[17, 24, 38]

184. B. The gestational sac in intrauterine pregnancy has two concentric outlines: an inner, complete outline and an outer, incomplete outline. These represent the decidua capsularis (inner) and the decidua parietalis, or vera (outer).[12, 33]

185. C. The diagnosis of microcephaly should only be made if the head circumference is more than 3 standard deviations below the mean. This assumes that the patient's dates are correct. Additional findings with microcephaly often include other congenital anomalies, such as hypo- or hypertelorism, limb malformations, and chromosomal abnormalities.[5, 12, 38]

186. B. Sonographic absence of a fluid-filled stomach over a 30- to 60-minute period of observation should raise the possibility of esophageal atresia. It may also be possible to demonstrate polyhydramnios. Esophageal atresia is sometimes seen in Down's syndrome and other chromosomal abnormalities. Fetuses should be closely examined for coexisting signs of such abnormalities.[5]

187. B. In the presence of a large allantoic cyst it is not uncommon to find all three of the cord vessels spread apart. Additionally, the um-

bilical vein, which is normally larger than the two umbilical arteries, may be compressed and smaller than expected. In most cases there is little clinical significance to most umbilical cord cysts (allantoic cysts); however, Fink and Filly noted an association between them and omphaloceles.[12, 23, 36, 47]

188. B. The differentiation of the ureters from the internal iliac veins can be achieved by observing that the ureters terminate bluntly into the bladder wall, whereas the iliac veins eventually bifurcate.[1, 67]

189. C. The Lippes Loop has a specific morphological pattern on sonography that allows one to identify them as to type in a high percentage of cases (94%). The Lippes Loop creates five interrupted echoes of moderate to high amplitude on longitudinal scans, representing the coils being transected by the beam.[1, 5, 12, 61]

190. B. Besides the history of one or more C-sections, the presence of a low *anterior* placental implantation or a placenta previa and the presence of focal exophytic masses (such as fibroids) are all risk factors.[12, 56] A simple mnemonic method of remembering the characteristics of the different types of abnormal placental implantations is *AIP: A* represents *accreta* and the abnormal *attachment* of the placenta because of the lack of decidua basalis between it and the myometrium. *I* represents *increta* and *invasion* of the myometrium by the placental tissues. *P* represents *percreta* and the *penetration* of the placenta through the myometrium and adjacent structures.[17]

191. C. Thanatophoric dwarfism probably represents the most common lethal skeletal dysplasia manifest antenatally. Approximately 14% of thanatophoric dwarfs have the cloverleaf skull deformity, a severely enlarged and trilobed head readily apparent on the antenatal sonogram. Although the cloverleaf skull malformation may occur in a variety of syndromes, it manifests only in short-limbed dwarfs who have either thanatophoric dysplasia or homozygous achondroplasia.[33, 47, 53]

192. C. When the abdominal contents such as stomach and bowel are herniated into the chest through a diaphragmatic defect, it results in pulmonary compression. Subsequently pulmonary hypoplasia occurs and is the primary cause of mortality.[33]

193. D. The most common abnormality of the umbilical cord is the single umbilical artery (SUA), found in 0.5 to 1.0% of pregnancies. The clinical significance of SUA is an association with other fetal malformations in 14% to 62% of cases. Since anomalous fetuses with SUA

tend to have multiple malformations involving multiple organ systems, detection of SUA and at least one other malformation may help predict the presence of additional anomalies, many of which may not be visible. The presence of SUA in association with other malformations also significantly increases the likelihood of an underlying chromosomal disorder.[5, 12, 47, 53]

194. A. Bladder exstrophy involves eversion of the bladder and a ureter outside of the body. A defect is present through the lower abdominal wall and the anterior wall of the urinary bladder. Urinary bladder fill does not occur because the bladder opens into the amniotic fluid. However, oligohydramnios does not occur, because the unobstructed ureters may empty directly into the amniotic fluid. Also, a "mass" that represents the empty, everted urinary bladder may be visualized.[33, 53]

195. B. The sonographer must systematically scan through the cervix looking carefully for two endocervical canals and measuring the width of the cervix. If the width of the cervix or uterus is much more than the normal 5 cm, the possibility of duplication (didelphic uterus) must be explored.[5]

196. B. With duodenal atresia prominent peristaltic waves can be seen in the stomach as is seen with bowel obstruction.[12, 48]

197. B. Unilateral or bilateral hydronephrosis is present in association with obstruction at the junction of the renal pelvis and ureter. The ureters and urinary bladder are unremarkable.[33, 47, 53]

198. D. The amniotic fluid index (AFI) measures the vertical height of amniotic fluid pockets in each of the four quadrants of the uterus. A normal fluid volume is estimated to be approximately 24 cm. More importantly, a finding of 5 cm or less is indicative of oligohydramnios, while findings of 25 cm or more indicate polyhydramnios.[5, 32]

199. A. The kidneys may be abnormally enlarged with some syndromes or diseases such as the Beckwith-Wiedeman syndrome or renal vein thrombosis. Beckwith-Wiedeman syndrome is a sporadically occurring syndrome resulting in macrosomia, macroglossia, large kidneys, omphalocele, and many other abnormalities.[58] Renal thrombosis (RVT) is a well-known entity in neonates that often presents with palpably enlarged kidney(s) and varying degrees of renal failure. One important cause of RVT is maternal diabetes.[5, 33, 53]

200. B. To be diagnostic, the fetal heart rate should be determined at the same time that the maternal pulse is palpated. The fetal heart rate is generally considered to be twice the rate of the maternal heart. Although the fetal heart rate is normally 120 to 160 beats per minute, tachycardia in the mother may confuse the findings.[37,46,56,66]

201. B. Fetal ascites, when not due to hydrops, is due to genitourinary system abnormalities. It is implicated in the development of the lax abdominal musculature of prune belly syndrome. In suspected prune belly syndrome, undulation of the anterior abdominal wall of the fetus can be demonstrated when the transducer is used to tap on the mother's abdominal wall.[5]

202. C. In both fetal serum and amniotic fluid the concentration of AFP is highest around week 13 of gestation. After 13 weeks, the levels in both fetal serum and amniotic fluid normally decrease rapidly in parallel fashion, whereas those in the maternal serum continue to rise until late in pregnancy.[5,9,12]

203. C. Chronic ectopic pregnancy is a form of *tubal* pregnancy in which growth of trophoblastic tissue early in gestation causes gradual disintegration of the tubal wall and slow or repeated episodes of hemorrhage. The presence of blood, trophoblastic tissue, and disrupted tubal tissue in the peritoneal cavity incites an inflammatory response, which seals off the area, creating a pelvic hematocele.[5]

204. D. The diagnostic conclusion was that there was a single, viable intrauterine pregnancy of approximately 16+ weeks gestation in the cephalic position. Incidentally noted was a maternal pelvic kidney—without evidence of hydronephrosis—on the right side. The left maternal kidney was noted to be in the normal position. (Courtesy of Nancy Wityk, Johns Hopkins School of Diagnostic Medical Sonography, Baltimore, Maryland.)

205. C. Nuchal cord. (Courtesy of Dayna Landru and Tracy Pfizenmaier, St. Francis Hospital School of Diagnostic Medical Sonography, Milwaukee, Wisconsin.)

206. B. Transvaginal scans demonstrated a mass in the cul-de-sac, measuring approximately 2.5 cm and containing a fetal pole and yolk sac. Fluid was also noted in the cul-de-sac. The uterus was seen in multiple views and showed evidence of a normal endometrial pattern without evidence of intrauterine pregnancy. The sonographic diagnosis was of ectopic pregnancy with free-fluid within the cul-

de-sac. (Courtesy of Lisa Elbert, Community College of Allegheny County, Monroeville, Pennsylvania.)

207. B. *Sonographic diagnosis:* A large 13.5 cm × 18.8 cm × 11.3 cm complex left adnexal mass with multiple internal septations is present. Serous or mucinous cystadenoma or cystadenocarcinoma cannot be excluded. *Pathology diagnosis:* mucinous cystadenocarcinoma of low malignant potential (borderline tumor). (Courtesy of Stephanie Ellingson, University of Iowa Hospitals and Clinics, Iowa City, Iowa.)

208. C. Cystic hygromas are multiseptate cystic masses that are often bilateral.[12, 33, 47]

209. B. The majority of cystic hygromas (approximately 80%) are located posterolaterally along the neck.[58]

210. A. Cystic hygromas are thought to represent dilated obstructed jugular lymph sacs, thus placing them in the general category of lymphangiomas.[53]

211. D. Cystic hygromas commonly occur in association with Turner's syndrome, where the manifestation of a webbed neck is thought by many to represent the resolution of a cystic hygroma during fetal life.[54]

212. C. No fetal heart activity is seen in the M-mode scan.

213. B. After 16 weeks' gestation, measurement of the lateral ventricle should not exceed 10 mm (1 cm).[47] (Courtesy of Linda Lang, Johns Hopkins, Baltimore, Maryland and Stacey Beck, Orange Coast College, Costa Mesa, California.)

214. D. Ultrasound revealed a normal uterus and an echogenic mass with some internal shadowing, on the right ovary. The mass measured 4 to 5 cm in diameter. The left ovary was normal. A small amount of free-fluid was seen around the mass. The ultrasound diagnosis was that of a dermoid cyst (cystic teratoma), which was confirmed by X-ray (Fig. 5-20) and subsequent surgery. (Courtesy of Benita Barthel, Ochsner Medical Foundation, New Orleans, Louisiana.)

215. B. The 11.8 cm × 3.3 cm × 9.7 cm echogenic mass in the left posterior-inferior aspect of the uterus was diagnosed as a subchorionic hematoma.

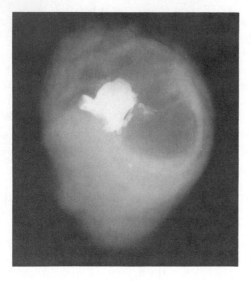

Figure 5-20. Radiograph: KUB.

216. C. It was felt that a myometrial contraction (Braxton-Hicks contraction) occurring at the time Figure 5-12*B* was obtained explains the diminished size of the subchorionic hematoma over the period of one week. (Courtesy of Anita Bowser, Community College of Allegheny County, Monroeville, Pennsylvania.)

217. D. The mucinous cystadenoma is an ovarian cyst characterized by a slightly lobulated appearance, gelatinous contents, and invariable multilocular nature due to the presence of numerous daughter cysts. They tend to become quite large.[24, 47] (Courtesy of Michelle Guillory, Ochsner Medical Foundation, New Orleans, Louisiana.)

218. C. Figure 5.14 demonstrates the presence of a cystic sac extending posterior from the sacrum. It appears to be continuous with the distal spinal canal, consistent with a lower lumbar sacral meningocele. No other anomalies were identified and lower extremity motion was demonstrated. (Courtesy of Bonnie S. Kazior, Community College of Allegheny County, Monroeville, Pennsylvania.)

219. C. The placenta was seen to cover the left anterolateral uterine wall. An additional "clump" of placenta was noted on the mid-posterior aspect of the uterine floor. Although the placenta is usually a single, discoid organ, one or more accessory lobes may occasionally develop, a condition called *placenta succenturiata*. The clinical importance of this condition is twofold: blood vessels connecting the accessory lobe to the placenta pass through the membranes

and can be torn during rupture of the membranes. And, an accessory lobe may not be delivered with the placenta, and retention within the uterus may cause serious hemorrhage.[46]

220. C. Ultrasound of the pelvis demonstrated an inhomogeneous, mostly hyperechoic mass in the left ovary measuring 7 cm × 3.9 cm × 3.4 cm in diameter. A similar mass with mostly hyperechoic components and some shadowing was seen in the right ovary, measuring 3.8 cm × 4.3 cm × 5.3 cm in diameter. The uterus is normal, and no pelvic fluid collections are seen. Impression: bilateral ovarian dermoid teratomas.

221. B. Water enemas may help differentiate a teratoma from bowel. In such procedures, the rectum is distended with 100 to 200 ml of lukewarm tap water introduced slowly. The microbubbles in the tap water provide sonographic "contrast," which helps to distinguish the rectum from the pelvic masses. The urinary bladder must be moderately distended for optimal visualization of pelvic structures with the water enema technique.[5,39] (Courtesy of Stephanie Ellingson, University of Iowa Hospitals and Clinics, Iowa City, Iowa.)

222. B. The clinical symptoms and age of this patient, coupled with the sonogram, make leiomyomatous uterus the most likely pathology. Since subserosal fibroids—even those attaining great size—are generally asymptomatic, the presence of submucous or intramural fibroids should be further investigated.[31]

223. A. While the transvaginal technique provides more detailed information about the architecture of the fibroid mass, the expanded field of view provided by transabdominal scans is needed to differentiate whether the mass is subserosal, submucous, or intramural in its location.[5,12,31]

224. D. Encephaloceles (encephalomeningoceles) result from failure of the surface ectoderm to separate from the neural ectoderm. This results in a bony calvarial defect that allows herniation of either the meninges alone or the brain and meninges.[47]

225. B. The most common site of occurrence is the occipital midline (75%), followed by the frontal midline (13%) and parietal (12%) locations.[47]

226. B. Among the other defects associated with encephalocele are Meckel's syndrome (encephalocele, microcephaly, polydactyly, cystic

kidneys), hydrocephalus, and Dandy-Walker syndrome.[12, 47] (Courtesy of Benita Barthel, Ochsner Medical Foundation, New Orleans, Louisiana.)

227. C. Transabdominal and transvaginal scans revealed the presence of an unruptured ectopic pregnancy in the right adnexal area. After a thorough examination of the left and right adnexa and failure to image the right ovary as separate from the gestational implant, the diagnosis of right ovarian ectopic pregnancy was made. According to Callen, 95% to 97% of ectopic pregnancies occur within the tube, with the ampullary portion of the tube the most common location. Ovarian ectopic pregnancy is a rare occurrence, accounting for only 1.5% to 1.0% of all ectopic gestations.[12, 47]

REFERENCES

1. Athey PA, Hadlock FP. Ultrasound in obstetrics and gynecology. 2nd ed. St. Louis: CV Mosby, 1985.
2. Austin K. Obstetrical pathology and complications. In: Guidelines for obstetrics and gynecology review. Dallas: Society of Diagnostic Medical Sonographers, 1990.
3. Benacerraf BY, Neuberg D, Bromley B, Frigoletto FD. Sonographic scoring index for prenatal detection of chromosomal abnormalities. J Ultrasound Med 1992; 11:449.
4. Benson CB, Coughlin BF, Doubilet PM. Amniotic fluid volume in large-for-gestational-age fetuses of nondiabetic mothers. J Ultrasound Med 1991;10:149.
5. Berman MC. Diagnostic medical sonography. Vol 1: Obstetrics and gynecology. Philadelphia: JB Lippincott, 1991.
6. Betz BW, Hertzberg BS, Carroll BA, Bowie JD. Mild fetal renal pelviectasis. J Ultrasound Med 1991;10:243.
7. Bromley B, Eslroff JA, Sanders SP, et al. Fetal echocardiography: accuracy and limitations in a population at high and low risk for heart defects. J Ultrasound Med 1992;11:S321.
8. Burke SR. Human anatomy and physiology for the health sciences. New York: John Wiley & Sons, 1980.
9. Burlbaw J. First trimester obstetrical ultrasound. In: Guidelines for obstetrics and gynecology review. Dallas: Society of Diagnostic Medical Sonographers, 1990.
10. Burton BK. Elevated maternal serum AFP: interpretation and follow-up. Clin Obstet Gynecol 1988;31:293.
11. Butler T, Kennedy L, Buttino L, Juberg RC. Prenatal sonographic renal findings associated with trisomy 13. J Diag Med Sonog 1992;8:262.
12. Callen PW. Ultrasonography in obstetrics and gynecology. 2nd ed. Philadelphia: WB Saunders, 1988.
13. Clark PK, Hurton TL, Stryker J, Benecerraf BR. Antenatal sonographic findings in trisomy 21. J Diag Med Sonog 1992;8:316.
14. Cohen HL. Pediatric and adolescent gynecologic ultrasound: normal, abnormal, and stimulators. J Ultrasound Med 1992;11:S30.
15. Comstock CH, Kirk DS. Arteriovenous malformations. J Ultrasound Med 1991; 10:361.
16. Craig M. Comprehensive obstetrical and gynecological sonography. Pleasanton, CA: Advanced Ultrasound Seminars, 1992.
17. Craig M. Pocket guide to ultrasound measurements. Philadelphia: JB Lippincott, 1988.
18. Drose J. Assessment of gestational age. In: Guidelines for obstetrics and gynecologic review. Dallas: Society of Diagnostic Medical Sonographers, 1990.
19. Drose J. The placenta. In: Guidelines for obstetrics and gynecologic review. Dallas: Society of Diagnostic Medical Sonographers, 1990.
20. Dubose TJ, Cunjus JA, Johnson LF. Normal embryo/fetal heart rates. J Ultrasound Med 1992;11:S22.
21. Finberg HJ, Williams JW. Placenta accreta: prospective sonographic diagnosis in patients with placenta previa and prior cesarean section. J Ultrasound Med 1992; 11:333.

22. Finberg HJ. Uterine synechiae in pregnancy: expanded criteria for recognition and review of clinical significance in 28 cases. J Ultrasound Med 1991;10:547.

23. Fink IJ, Filly RA. Omphalocele associated with umbilical cord allantoic cyst. Radiology 1983;149:473.

24. Fleischer AC, Jeanty P, James AE, et al. Principles and practice of ultrasonography in obstetrics and gynecology. 4th ed. East Norwalk, CT: Appleton & Lange, 1991.

25. Fleischer AC, Kepple DM. Transvaginal sonography. Philadelphia: JB Lippincott, 1992.

26. Goldstein SR, Snyder JR. Significance of presence or absence of cardiac activity by endovaginal ultrasound in very early pregnancy. J Ultrasound Med 1992;11:S22.

27. Goldstein SR. Subchorionic bleeding in threatened abortion: sonographic findings and significance. Am J Roentgenol 1983;141:975.

28. Granberg S, Wikland M, Karlson B, et al. Endometrial thickness as measured by endovaginal ultrasonography for identifying endometrial abnormality. Am J Obstet Gynecol 1991;164:47.

29. Gray DL, Crane JP. Selection of optimal nuchal skinfold thickening based on gestational age as a screen for Down's syndrome. J Ultra Med 1992;11:S39.

30. Gray P, Rouse GA, DeLange M. Sonographic evaluation of twin embolization syndrome. J Diag Med Sonog 1993;9:3.

31. Green TH. Gynecology: essentials of clinical practice. 3rd ed. Boston: Little Brown, 1977.

32. Hall R. The ultrasound handbook. Philadelphia: JB Lippincott, 1988.

33. Hegge FN. A practical guide to ultrasound of fetal anomalies. New York: Raven Press, 1992.

34. Heisterman J, Filly RA, Goldstin RB. Effect of measurement errors on sonography: evaluation of ventriculomegaly. J Ultrasound Med 1991;10:121.

35. Hertzberg BS, Bowie JD. Ultrasound of the postpartum uterus. J Ultrasound Med 1991;10:451.

36. Hsieh, F-J, Chen H-F, Ko T-M, et al. Antenatal diagnosis of vasa previa by color-flow mapping. J Ultrasound Med 1991;10:397.

37. Humes RA. Evaluation of fetal arrhythmias. J Ultrasound Med 1992;11:S4.

38. Jeanty P, Romero R. Obstetrical ultrasound. New York: McGraw-Hill, 1984.

39. Kawamura D. Patient care and preparation. In: Guidelines for obstetrics and gynecology review. Dallas: Society of Diagnostic Medical Sonographers, 1990.

40. Kawamura D. Pelvic anatomy. In: Guidelines for obstetric and gynecologic review. Dallas: Society of Diagnostic Medical Sonographers, 1990.

41. Kawamura D. Scanning techniques. In: Guidelines for obstetric and gynecologic review. Dallas: Society of Diagnostic Medical Sonographers, 1990.

42. Merchline M. Association of juvenile hypothyroidism and cystic ovaries. Radiology 1981;139(1):77.

43. Moore KL. The developing human. 2nd ed. Philadelphia: WB Saunders, 1977.

44. Moore TR. Ultrasound helps detection of fetal growth disorders. Diagnostic Imaging, 1989;April:122.

45. Netter FH. The Ciba collection of medical illustrations. Vol 1: The reproductive system. Summit, NJ: CIBA Geigy, 1965.

46. Niswander KR. Obstetrics: essentials of clinical practice. Boston: Little Brown, 1977.

47. Nyberg DA. Diagnostic ultrasound of fetal anomalies: text and atlas. Chicago: Yearbook, 1990.

48. Paulson EK, Hertzberg BS. Hyperechoic meconium in the third trimester fetus: an uncommon normal variant. J Ultrasound Med 1991;10:677.

49. Pena AJ, Schorr SJ, Corlon SJ, Rath L. Gartner's duct cyst described by endovaginal ultrasound. J Diag Med Sonog 1992;8:323.

50. Rabinowitz R, Peters M, Vyas S, et al. Measurement of fetal urine production in normal pregnancy by real-time ultrasonography. Am J Obstet Gynecol 1989;161:1264.

51. Robbins S. Pathological basis of disease. 3rd ed. Philadelphia: WB Saunders, 1987.

52. Rodis J, Vinzeleos A, Campbell W, et al. Intrauterine fetal growth in discordant twin gestations. J Ultrasound Med 1990;9:443.

53. Romero R, Pilu G, Jeanty P. Prenatal diagnosis of congenital anomalies. East Norwalk, CT: Appleton & Lange, 1988.

54. Rumack CM, Wilson SR, Charboneau JW. Diagnostic ultrasound. Vol 2: Obstetrics and pediatrics. St. Louis: Mosby-Yearbook, 1991.

55. Russel JB. The etiology of ectopic pregnancy. Clin Obstet Gynecol 1987;30:183.

56. Sabbagha RE. Diagnostic ultrasound applied to obstetrics and gynecology. 2nd ed. Philadelphia: JB Lippincott, 1987.

57. Sanders RC. Clinical sonography: a practical guide. Boston: Little Brown, 1984.

58. Sarti DA. Diagnostic ultrasound: text and cases. 2nd ed. Chicago: Year Book Medical Publishers, 1987.

59. Sauerbrei EE, Nguyen KT, Nolan RT. Abdominal sonography. New York: Raven Press, 1992.

60. Saw PD, Rouse GA, DeLange M. Meckel syndrome: sonographic findings. J Diag Med Sonog 1991;7:8.

61. Seagraves M. Gynecology. In: Guidelines for obstetrics and gynecology review. Dallas: Society of Diagnostic Medical Sonographers, 1990.

62. Sherer DM, Abramowicz JS, Thompson HO, et al. Comparison of transabdominal and endovaginal sonographic approaches in the diagnosis of a case of cervical pregnancy successfully treated with Methotrexate. J Ultrasound Med 1991;10:409.

63. Sherer DM, Hearn B, Abramowicz JS. Echogenic oral labial fissure: an aid to ruling out fetal cleft lip. J Ultrasound Med 1991;10:239.

64. Sherer DM, Roberts D, Rideout J, et al. Preoperative endovaginal sonographic diagnosis of an unruptured interstitial pregnancy. J Diag Med Sonog 1992;8:203.

65. Sherer DM, Smith SA, Allen T, et al. Sonographic diagnosis of a viable ampullary tubal pregnancy at 14 weeks' gestation. J Diag Med Sonog 1991;7:12.

66. Smith C, Grube GL, Wilson S. Maternal alpha-fetoprotein screening and the role of ultrasound. J Diag Med Sonog 1990;6:312.

67. Snell RS. Clinical embryology for medical students. 2nd ed. Boston: Little Brown, 1972.

68. Stamm E, Waldstein G, Thickman D, McGregor J. Amniotic sheets: natural history and histology. J Ultrasound Med 1991;10:501.

69. Thomas RS, Peng CC, Eglinton GS, et al. Precision of umbilical artery Doppler studies. J Ultrasound Med 1991;10:201.

70. Zilanti M, Azuaga A, Calderon F, et al. Transperineal sonography in second trimester to term pregnancies and early labor. J Ultrasound Med 1991;10:481.

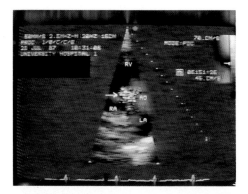

Plate 6-1. Short-axis basilar view, selective color map.

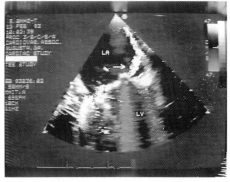

Plate 6-2. Transesophageal view of the left atrium and ventricle.

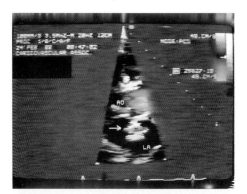

Plate 6-3. Two-dimensional superimposed color map (long axis).

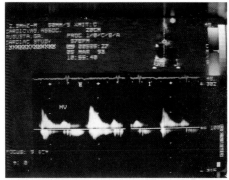

Plate 6-4. Color-flow, directed, pulsed-wave Doppler.

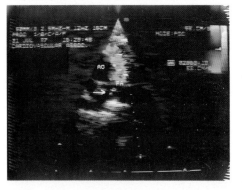

Plate 6-5. Short axis two-dimensional image with color-flow Doppler.

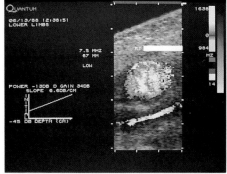

Plate 7-1. Groin mass.

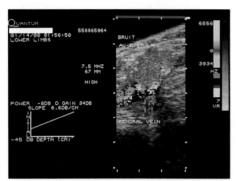

Plate 7-2. Doppler study of a Dale shunt. (Courtesy of David E. Smith, M.D., Good Samaritan Hospital, San Jose, California.)

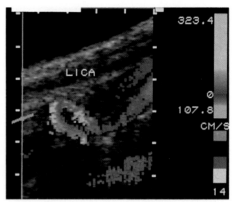

Plate 7-3. Carotid artery color-flow scan. (Courtesy of Richard W. Starrett, Good Samaritan Hospital, San Jose, California.)

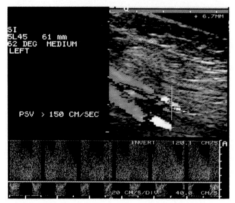

Plate 7-4. Scan of the lower extremity. (Courtesy of Roger Hayashi, M.D., Good Samaritan Hospital, San Jose, California.)

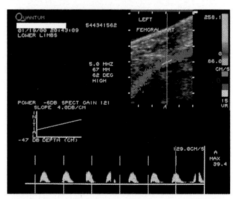

Plate 7-5. Femoral artery Doppler spectral analysis.

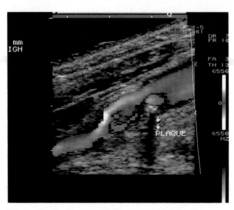

Plate 7-6. Scan of the carotid bulb.

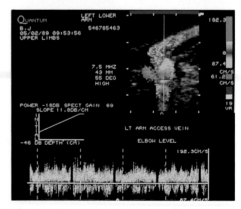

Plate 7-7. Access vein color flow.

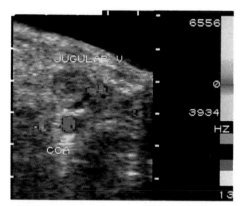

Plate 7-8. Carotid artery and jugular vein scan.

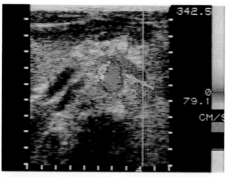

Plate 7-9. Left renal artery.

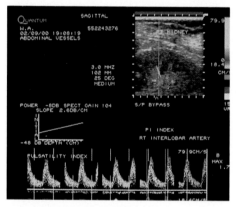

Plate 7-10. Renal interlobar arteries.

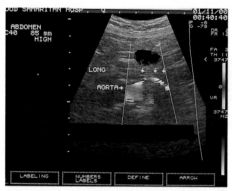

Plate 7-11. Longitudinal scan of the terminal aorta.

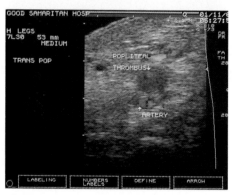

Plate 7-12. Venous lower extremity scan.

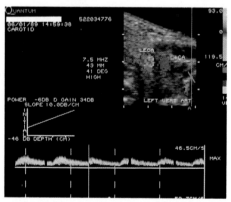

Plate 7-13. Transverse cross-sectional color-flow scan.

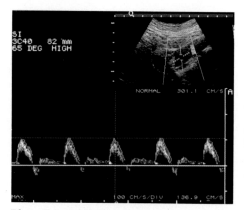

Plate 7-14. Aortic scan.

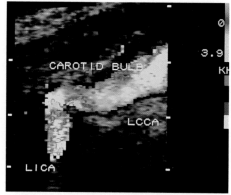

Plate 7-15. Internal carotid artery.

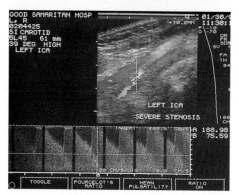

Plate 7-16. Stenotic waveform.

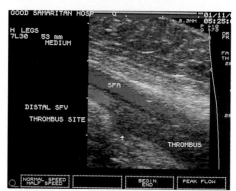

Plate 7-17. Lower extremity color-flow scan.

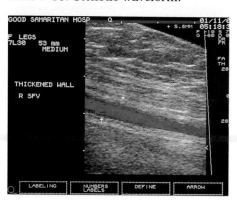

Plate 7-18. Venous study.

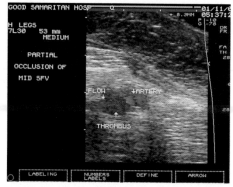

Plate 7-19. Superficial femoral vein scan.

Marveen Craig: *Ultrasound Exam Review*, © 1994 J. B. Lippincott Co.

6

JOHN CHARLES POPE

Echocardiography

OBJECTIVES

Although echocardiography is a relative newcomer to the field of diagnostic ultrasound, major technologic advances have produced rapid utilization of the technique in clinical medicine. M-mode echocardiography developed in the 1960s, and, used as an investigational tool in the mid-1970s, became the cornerstone of the echo exam in the late '70s. It was replaced by the two-dimensional examination in the early '80s, followed by pulsed and continuous-wave Doppler. The addition of color-flow Doppler propelled the simultaneous use of two-dimensional imaging with color flow superimposed information.

In short, this powerful noninvasive tool developed rapidly over several decades. Two-dimensional echo-Doppler examinations are now an essential part of any cardiac evaluation, whether it be congenital heart disease, valvular disease, or coronary artery disease. The purpose of this chapter is to prepare the reader for the wide variety of important clinical applications of these techniques in both registry examination and practical clinical settings.

QUESTIONS

Directions

Each of the questions or incomplete statements is followed by several answers or completions. Select the best answer(s) in each case. In the matching sections, answers should be used only once, unless otherwise stated.

1. In normal patients, the posterior mitral valve leaflet:
   A. moves in the same direction as the anterior leaflet.
   B. "mirrors" the anterior leaflet.
   C. moves paradoxically to the anterior leaflet.
   D. A and C

2. On an M-mode tracing, an E-F slope velocity of less than 15 mm/s suggests:
   A. severe mitral stenosis.
   B. mild mitral stenosis.
   C. moderate mitral stenosis.
   D. none of the above

3. The portion of the right ventricle that leads into the pulmonary artery is called the:
   A. *trabeculae.*
   B. *orifice.*
   C. *chordae tendinae.*
   D. *infundibulum.*

4. Aortic insufficiency (AI) may be caused by:
   A. aortic root dilatation.
   B. aortic regurgitation.
   C. rheumatic fever.
   D. A and C

5. The sinus of Valsalva is also known as the:
   A. coronary cusp.
   B. truncus arteriosus.
   C. aortic annulus.
   D. coronary sinus.

6. Mitral valve motion responds to all of the following *except:*
   A. left atrial pressure.
   B. left ventricular pressure.
   C. aortic pressure.
   D. pulmonic pressure.

7. Which of the following conditions is associated with exaggerated left ventricular posterior wall (LVPW) motion and poor septal motion?
   A. Aortic insufficiency
   B. Cardiomyopathy
   C. Coronary artery disease
   D. Myxoma

8. When performing mitral valve phonocardiogram studies, the initial vibrations of the first heart sound will occur simultaneously with the _____ point of the mitral valve.
   A. E
   B. C
   C. R
   D. A

9. Which of the following characteristics of the heart is *incorrect?*
   A. Acts as a double pump
   B. The right side handles deoxygenated blood
   C. The left side handles oxygenated blood
   D. The right and left atrial and ventricular cavities communicate

10. Patients with emphysema are best scanned from the _____ approach.
    A. suprasternal
    B. parasternal
    C. apical
    D. subcostal

11. Another term used to describe the epicardium is the _____ *layer:*
    A. *fibrous*
    B. *membranous*
    C. *parietal*
    D. *visceral*

12. Demonstration of a "swinging heart" should prompt investigation of the:
    A. pericardial sac.
    B. right ventricle.
    C. mitral valve.
    D. posterior wall of the left ventricle.

13. When ventricular pressure falls below atrial pressure, which of the following events occur(s)?
    A. Intake valves open
    B. The filling phase begins
    C. Ventricular contraction ceases
    D. All of the above

14. Patients with alcoholic cardiomyopathy often demonstrate:
    A. left ventricular enlargement.
    B. thinning of the interventricular septum.
    C. thickening of the left posterior ventricular wall.
    D. A and B

15. The left atrium provides openings for _____ pulmonary vein(s).

A. one
B. two
C. three
D. four

16. Patients with Marfan's syndrome generally exhibit all of the following findings *except:*
    A. aortic insufficiency.
    B. atrophy of the aortic root.
    C. pulmonary artery dilatation.
    D. B and C

17. The coronary sulcus is also known as the _____ groove.
    A. atrioventricular
    B. trilateral
    C. terminal
    D. interventricular

18. Which of the following events occur(s) during ventricular systole?
    A. The aortic valve opens
    B. The pulmonic valve is open
    C. The mitral valve is closed
    D. All of the above

19. The left ventricular outflow tract is separated by the:
    A. mitral annulus.
    B. anterior leaflet of the mitral valve.
    C. interventricular septum.
    D. aortic root.

20. Another term used to describe the coronary valve is the:
    A. *thebesian valve.*
    B. *valvulae conniventes.*
    C. *limbic valve.*
    D. *bicuspid valve.*

21. Maximum opening of the mi-

tral valve is usually indicated
by the:

A. A point.
B. C point.
C. E point.
D. F point.

22. The relationship of the pulmonary valve to the aortic root can be described as:

A. anterior and lateral.
B. superior and lateral.
C. posterior and medial.
D. inferior and medial.

23. Which of the following is (are) *not* considered part of the circulatory system?

A. Cardiovascular apparatus
B. Lymphatic system
C. Blood-forming and blood-destroying tissues
D. Cardiac-governing nerves and hormones

24. Blood flows from the lungs via the pulmonary veins to the:

A. right atrium.
B. left atrium.
C. right ventricle.
D. left ventricle.

25. The first heart sound is associated with:

A. AV valve closure and semilunar valve opening.
B. AV valve opening and semilunar valve closure.
C. AV valve opening and semilunar valve opening.
D. A and C

26. The companion vein to the left coronary artery is the:

A. great cardiac vein.
B. lesser cardiac vein.

C. middle cardiac vein.
D. superior cardiac vein.

27. The ejection phase begins:

A. when the atrial pressure rises.
B. when the ventricular pressure exceeds aortic, pulmonic, and atrial pressures.
C. with myocardial relaxation.
D. A and C

28. The small mass of specialized myocardial cells embedded in the right atrial wall near the entrance of the superior vena cava is known as the:

A. bundle of His.
B. AV node.
C. SA node.
D. Purkinje cluster.

29. The cardiac cycle consists of systolic (contracting) movement and a diastolic (filling) movement. Of the two, _____ lasts almost twice as long as

_____ .

A. diastole; systole
B. systole; diastole
C. ventricular contraction; atrial filling
D. none of the above

30. The right atrioventricular opening is also known as the:

A. mitral orifice.
B. tricuspid orifice.
C. aortic orifice.
D. pulmonic orifice.

31. Compared to the right ventricle, the left ventricle:

A. has thinner walls.
B. is longer and narrower.

C. is shorter and wider.
D. has weaker papillary muscle tone.

Match the correct definitions to numbers 32–41.

A. Rolling or turning inward; regression of tissue without degeneration
B. "Hollowed" breast
C. Clot formation
D. Line of union of the halves of various symmetrical parts
E. Tissue death
F. Necrotic tissue coagulation resulting from circulatory occlusion
G. Closure; obstruction or closing off
H. Union of corresponding parts
I. Yielding to pressure or force without destruction
J. Fragmentary or incomplete or paradoxical movement

32. ___ Necrosis
33. ___ Thrombosis
34. ___ Occlusion
35. ___ Involution
36. ___ Infarct
37. ___ Compliance
38. ___ Pectus excavatum
39. ___ Commissure
40. ___ Dyskinesia
41. ___ Raphe

42. Select the term used to describe an unusual prolonged conduction route in which the cardiac impulse always meets an area that is no longer refractory and thus keeps traveling around the heart.

A. Circuit movement
B. Circus movement
C. Disorganized contraction
D. Fibrillation

43. The cardiovascular system can be subdivided into two systems:
A. arterial and venous.
B. pulmonic and systemic.
C. hematologic and lymphatic.
D. B and C

44. Which of the following activities precede(s) ventricular systole?
A. Ventricular depolarization waves
B. Rising ventricular pressure
C. AV valve opening
D. A and B

45. Which of the following statements about the right pulmonary artery is (are) *false?*
A. It is longer than the left pulmonary artery
B. It is shorter than the left pulmonary artery
C. It divides into two primary branches
D. B and C

46. The total volumes of blood pumped through the pulmonary and systemic circuits in a given period of time are:
A. staggered.
B. equal.
C. unequal.
D. A and C

47. Stimulation of the parasympathetic fibers to the SA node will result in a (an):
A. increased heart rate.

B. decreased heart rate.
C. irregular heart rate.
D. stable heart rate.

48. The aortic and pulmonary semilunar valves have a combined total of _____ cusps.
    A. two
    B. four
    C. six
    D. eight

49. Thin fibrous bands, called chordae tendinae, attach to:
    A. each cusp of the two atrioventricular valves.
    B. the papillary muscle.
    C. the mitral valve ring.
    D. A and C

50. The "P" wave of an electrocardiogram corresponds to:
    A. AV node firing.
    B. SA node firing.
    C. atrial expansion.
    D. ventricular filling.

51. Auscultation of the pulmonary valve is best achieved at the:
    A. second right intercostal space.
    B. third left costal cartilage.
    C. fourth costal cartilage.
    D. fifth intercostal space.

52. All of the following findings are seen in patients with hypertrophic cardiomyopathy *except:*
    A. increased left ventricular size and volume.
    B. systolic pressure gradients cross the left ventricular outflow tract.
    C. morphologic changes in the interventricular septum.
    D. A and C

53. Ebstein's anomaly is characterized by:
    A. prolapse of the mitral valve.
    B. excessive motion or malposition of the tricuspid valve
    C. IHSS.
    D. pulmonic stenosis.

54. Which of the following is classified as mechanical, ball-and-cage prosthetic valves?
    A. Bjork-Shiley
    B. Carpentier-Edwards
    C. St. Jude
    D. Starr-Edwards

55. The combination of increased venous pressure, decreased systemic blood pressure, and quiet heart occurs in acute tamponade due to intrapericardial bleeding. This constellation of findings is commonly known as:
    A. Austin's triad.
    B. Beck's triad.
    C. Danforth's triad.
    D. Loeffler's triad.

56. Which of the following statements concerning cor triatrium is *untrue?*
    A. Fails to incorporate the embryonic common pulmonary vein into the left atrium
    B. Pulmonary veins empty into an accessory chamber inferior to the true left atrium
    C. Demonstrates turbulent, high-velocity flow proximal to the mitral valve
    D. Results in obstructed pulmonary venous flow

CASES AND QUESTIONS

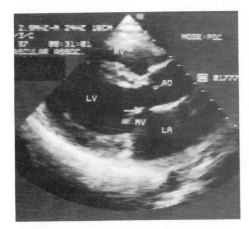

Figure 6-1. Parasternal long-axis view.

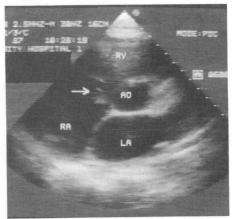

Figure 6-2. Parasternal short-axis view, basilar section.

57. Name the most likely defect indicated by the arrow in this two-dimensional scan (Fig. 6-1).
    A. Mitral valve prolapse
    B. Artifact produced by poor interrogation angle
    C. Cleft mitral valve leaflet
    D. Mitral valve stenosis

58. An additional abnormality commonly associated with this defect is:
    A. muscular ventricular septal defect.
    B. mitral valve regurgitation.
    C. ostium primum atrial septal defect.
    D. ostium secundum atrial septal defect.

59. This 35-year-old patient complained of increasing dyspnea. The echocardiogram (Fig. 6-2) is suspicious for:
    A. tricuspid valve vegetation.
    B. a right atrial tumor.
    C. rupture of the sinus of Valsalva.
    D. network of Chiari.

60. The color-flow Doppler study in Plate 6-1 reveals:
    A. turbulent flow consistent with atrial septal defect.
    B. turbulent flow consistent with aortic right atrial fistula.
    C. turbulent flow consistent with tricuspid valve regurgitation.
    D. nonspecific right atrial flow pattern.

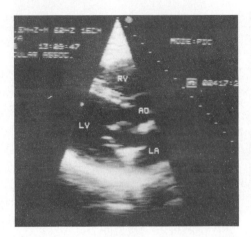

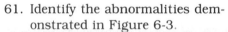

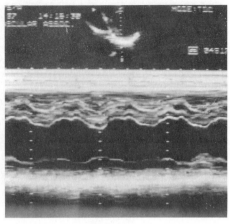

Figure 6-3. Two-dimensional long-axis view.

Figure 6-4. M-mode tracing: mid-ventricular level.

61. Identify the abnormalities demonstrated in Figure 6-3.
    1. Calcified mitral valve leaflets
    2. Enlarged right ventricle
    3. Restricted mitral valve motion
    4. Mitral annular calcification
    5. Thickened pericardium
    A. 1 and 4
    B. 2 and 4
    C. 1, 2, and 5
    D. 1, 3, and 4

62. If the mitral valve pressure half-time is 172 m/s, the mitral valve orifice is:
    A. 1.3 cm^2.
    B. 1.4 cm^2.
    C. 0.9 cm^2.
    D. 1.0 cm^2.

63. This 72-year-old patient is being evaluated for chest discomfort. His EKG is within normal limits. The M-mode echocardiogram (Fig. 6-4) reveals:
    A. anteroseptal myocardial infarction.
    B. constrictive pericarditis.
    C. left ventricular enlargement.
    D. posterior myocardial infarction.

64. The Doppler abnormality associated with Figure 6-4 would most likely be:
    A. increased mitral inflow A component due to diastolic abnormality.
    B. mitral inflow E point variable amplitude related to respiratory dependency.
    C. mitral valve regurgitation.
    D. aortic valve regurgitation.

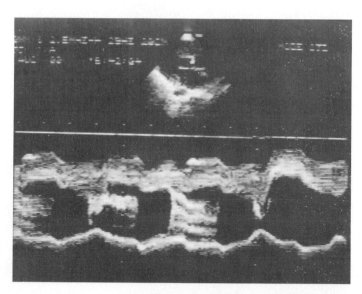

Figure 6-5. M-mode sweep proximal to the aortic root.

65. This M-mode recording (Fig. 6-5) is consistent with:
    A. mitral valve mass.
    B. shaggy echoes prolapsing into the left ventricular out-flow tract.
    C. abnormal interventricular septal motion.
    D. left atrial mass.

66. The abnormality demonstrated in Figure 6-5 is consistent with:
    A. vegetation due to endocarditis.
    B. thrombus.
    C. IHSS.
    D. myxoma.

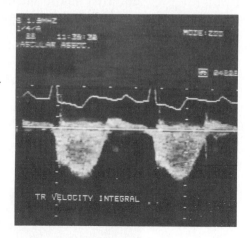

Figure 6-6. Continuous-wave Doppler tracing.

67. Calculate the pulmonic arterial systolic pressure from the tricuspid velocity integral presented in Figure 6-6.
    A. 25 mm/hg
    B. 35 mm/hg
    C. 50 mm/hg
    D. 90 mm/hg

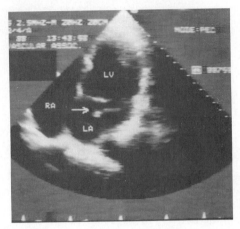

Figure 6-7. Modified apical four-chamber view.

68. This apical four-chamber view (Fig. 6-7) is consistent with:
    1. enlarged left ventricle.
    2. atrial septal defect.
    3. enlarged left atrium.
    4. flail mitral valve leaflet.
    A. 1 and 4
    B. 2 and 3
    C. 1, 2, and 3
    D. 1, 3, and 4

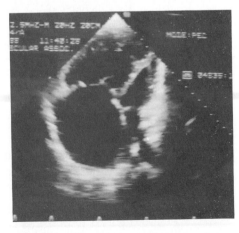

Figure 6-8. Two-dimensional apical view.

69. The most likely defect associated with this two-dimensional echocardiogram (Fig. 6-8) is:
    A. tricuspid valve atresia.
    B. atrial septal defect.
    C. pulmonary embolus.
    D. ventricular septal defect.

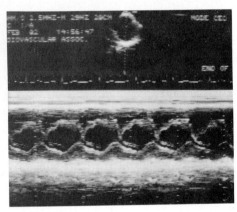

Figure 6-9. M-mode scan of mid-right and left ventricle.

70. Associated abnormalities seen in Figure 6-9 are:
    1. early diastolic septal notching.
    2. left bundle branch block pattern of septal motion.
    3. hyperdynamic septal motion.
    4. marked cyclic ventricular size variation.
    A. 1 and 4
    B. 2 and 4
    C. 3 and 4
    D. 1 and 3

71. Pericardial effusion causes separation of the:
    A. myocardium from the epicardium.
    B. endocardium from the visceral pericardium.

C. epicardium from the parietal pericardium.

D. visceral pericardium from the epicardium.

72. Paradoxical septal motion may be caused by:
    1. right bundle branch block.
    2. acute pulmonary embolus.
    3. mitral valve regurgitation.
    4. atrial septal defect.
    A. 1 and 3
    B. 2 and 4
    C. 1 and 2
    D. 2 and 3

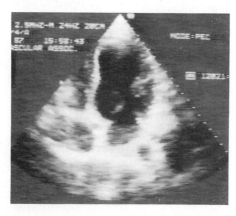

Figure 6-10. Modified left ventricular apical view.

73. The most significant abnormalities in Figure 6-10 are:
    1. anteroseptal wall thinning and scar.
    2. apical thrombus.
    3. probably left ventricular dysfunction.
    4. a thickened pericardium.
    A. 1 and 3
    B. 2 and 4
    C. 1 and 2
    D. 2 and 3

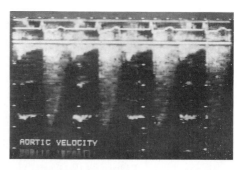

Figure 6-11. Continuous-wave Doppler tracing.

74. Calculate the aortic valve peak gradient from the Doppler velocity in Figure 6-11.
    A. 36 mm/hg
    B. 50 mm/hg
    C. 64 mm/hg
    D. 70 mm/hg

75. Calculate the aortic valve orifice using the velocity above, with an LVOT equaling 2.0 cm and an LVOTV equaling 100 cm/s.
    A. 0.9 cm^2
    B. 1.0 cm^2
    C. .78 cm^2
    D. .85 cm^2

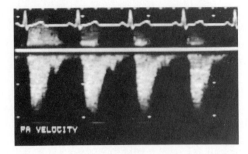

Figure 6-12. Continuous-wave Doppler tracing of pulmonary artery.

76. The Doppler velocity in Figure 6-12 corresponds to:
    A. mild pulmonic stenosis.
    B. normal pulmonic flow.
    C. severe pulmonic stenosis.
    D. moderate pulmonic stenosis.

77. Papillary muscle dysfunction is commonly seen in:
    A. congestive heart failure.
    B. ischemic heart disease.
    C. hypertrophic cardiomyopathy.
    D. mitral valve prolapse.

78. Complications of myocardial infarction include:
    1. congestive heart failure.
    2. recurrent angina pectoris.
    3. cardiac arrhythmias.
    4. aortic regurgitation.
    A. 1 and 3
    B. 2 and 4
    C. 1, 2, and 3
    D. 2, 3, and 4

79. Indications for transesophageal echocardiography include:
    1. evaluation of left ventricular function.
    2. search for embolic source.
    3. valvular heart disease.
    4. investigation for valvular vegetation.
    A. 1 and 3
    B. 2 and 4
    C. 1, 2, and 3
    D. 2, 3, and 4

80. The transesophageal echocardiogram in Plate 6-2 is consistent with:
    A. prosthetic valve dysfunction with mild mitral valve regurgitation.
    B. normal prosthetic valve function with mild regurgitation.
    C. mitral valve regurgitation secondary to rheumatic valvular heart disease.
    D. moderate mitral valve regurgitation related to mitral valve prosthetic dysfunction.

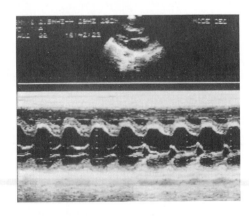

Figure 6-13. M-mode scan of the proximal and mid-left ventricle.

81. The M-mode echocardiogram in Figure 6-13 is most consistent with:
    A. posterior wall myocardial infarction.

B. mitral valve regurgitation with left ventricular volume overload.

C. left ventricular volume overload with early mitral valve closure.

D. congestive cardiomyopathy.

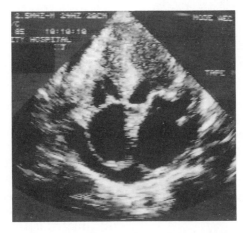

Figure 6-14. Four-chamber apical view.

82. The two-dimensional echocardiogram in Figure 6-14 is consistent with:
    A. pericardial effusion.
    B. infiltrative cardiomyopathy.
    C. left ventricular hypertrophy.
    D. restrictive cardiomyopathy.

83. The color-flow Doppler in Plate 6-3 most likely represents:
    A. mitral valve regurgitation.
    B. aortic valve regurgitation.
    C. aortic left atrial fistula.
    D. artifact.

84. The following characteristics may be seen with a "swinging heart":
    1. right ventricular enlargement.
    2. right atrial collapse.
    3. systolic anterior motion of the mitral valve.
    4. paradoxical motion of the intraventricular septum.
    A. 1 and 3
    B. 2 and 4
    C. 1, 2, and 3
    D. 2, 3, and 4

85. The most common metastatic tumor of the heart is a:
    A. melanoma.
    B. fibroma.
    C. rhabdomyoma.
    D. sarcoma.

86. The most common primary cardiac malignancy is a:
    A. rhabdomyoma.
    B. sarcoma.
    C. myxoma.
    D. angiosarcoma.

87. An arterial embolus may be traced to:
    1. left ventricular mural thrombus.
    2. left atrial appendage mass.
    3. right ventricular thrombus.
    4. venous thrombus in the presence of a patent foramen ovale.
    A. 1 and 4
    B. 2 and 4
    C. 1, 2, and 4
    D. 2, 3, and 4

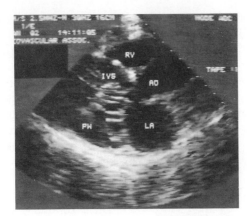

Figure 6-15. Two-dimensional parasternal long-axis view.

88. The two-dimensional echocardiogram in Figure 6-15 is consistent with:
    A. left ventricular hypertrophy.
    B. right ventricular hypertrophy.
    C. IHSS.
    D. infiltrative cardiomyopathy.

89. Characteristic M-mode findings of hypertrophic cardiomyopathy include:
    1. right ventricular hypertrophy.
    2. asymmetrical septal hypertrophy.
    3. aortic valve stenosis.
    4. systolic anterior motion of the mitral valve.

5. mitral valve regurgitation.
    A. 2 and 3
    B. 2 and 4
    C. 2, 4, and 5
    D. 1, 3, and 5

90. The second heart sound is produced by the:
    A. closing of the atrioventricular valves.
    B. closing of the semilunar valves.
    C. opening of the semilunar valves.
    D. opening of the atrioventricular valves.

91. The M-mode pattern of dilated cardiomyopathy consists of:
    1. normal right ventricular dimension and contractility.
    2. dilated left ventricular cavity.
    3. normal left ventricular fractional shortening.
    4. diminished left ventricular fractional shortening.
    5. diminished excursion of the aortic valve.
    A. 2 and 3
    B. 2 and 4
    C. 2, 4, and 5
    D. 1, 3, and 5

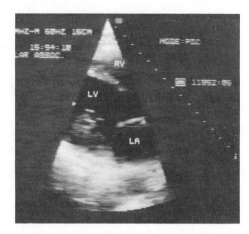

Figure 6-16. Parasternal long-axis view.

92. The occluded coronary artery involved in Figure 6-16 is the:
    A. right coronary artery.
    B. circumflex coronary artery.
    C. left anterior descending coronary artery.
    D. obtuse marginal coronary artery.

93. When a patient with known diastolic dysfunction presents with a normal Doppler mitral inflow integral tracing, the most likely explanation is:
    A. the presence of mitral regurgitation.
    B. reversion to restrictive diastolic function.
    C. pseudo-normalization of the Doppler tracing.
    D. that the Doppler is not a reliable indicator of diastolic function.

Match the correct pressure with the appropriate anatomical structure in numbers 94–99.

A. 3–12 mm/hg end diastolic
B. 70–105 mm/hg mean
C. 1–10 mm/hg mean diastolic
D. 0–8 mm/hg end diastolic
E. 16–30 mm/hg peak systolic
F. 2–10 mm/hg A wave

94. ___ Right atrium
95. ___ Right ventricle
96. ___ Left atrium
97. ___ Left ventricle
98. ___ Pulmonary artery
99. ___ Systemic artery

100. Normal oxygen saturation for the right ventricle is:
    A. 98%.
    B. 70%.
    C. 80%.
    D. 75%.

Match the appropriate left ventricular formulae with the definitions in numbers 101–106.

A. (LVPWs − LVPWd) ÷ (LVPWd) × 100
B. (EDV − ESV) ÷ (EDV) × 100
C. (IVSs − IVSd ÷ IVSd) × 100
D. (LVIDd − LVIDs ÷ LVIDd) × 100
E. (LVIDd − LVIDs) ÷ (LVIDd) × LVET)
F. 1.04 (IVSd + PWLVd + LVIDd)^3 − (LVIDd)^3 − 13.6 gm

101. ___ Interventricular septal percent thickening
102. ___ Left ventricular posterior wall percent thickening
103. ___ Left ventricular fractional shortening

104. ___ Left ventricular ejection fraction
105. ___ Left ventricular mass
106. ___ Mean VcF

107. A jet height/left ventricular outflow tract measurement of 45% is considered:
    A. moderate aortic regurgitation.
    B. mild aortic regurgitation.
    C. severe aortic regurgitation.
    D. moderately severe aortic regurgitation.

108. Systolic reversal of pulmonic vein flow seen during transesophageal echocardiographic examination is consistent with:
    A. a normal finding.
    B. mild mitral valve regurgitation.
    C. pseudo-normalization of diastolic function.
    D. moderate to severe mitral valve regurgitation.

109. A Stage III left ventricular diastolic filling pattern reveals:
    1. an E-A ratio less than 1.5.
    2. a deceleration time greater than 240 m/s.
    3. IVRT less than 60 m/s.
    4. pulmonary vein A wave reversal less than 25 cm/s.
    5. deceleration time of less than 160 m/s.
    A. 1, 2, and 3
    B. 2 and 4
    C. 3 and 5
    D. 3, 4, and 5

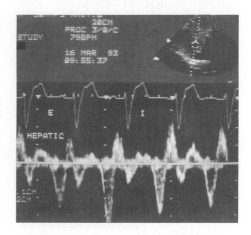

Figure 6-17. Pulsed-wave hepatic vein recording.

110. The Doppler tracing in Figure 6-17 is most consistent with:
    A. normal flow.
    B. constrictive pericarditis.
    C. intravascular volume overload.
    D. restrictive myocardial disease.

111. A transesophageal mitral regurgitant jet area of 4 cm^2 is consistent with:
    A. mild mitral valve regurgitation.
    B. moderately severe mitral valve regurgitation.
    C. moderate mitral valve regurgitation.
    D. severe mitral valve regurgitation.

112. Clockwise rotation of a biplane transesophageal probe longitudinally to the most medial position will allow visualization of:
    A. two-chamber view of left atrium and left ventricle.
    B. short-axis view of the

    aorta and the right ventricular inflow and outflow tracts.
- C. the right atrium and connections to superior vena cava and an inferior vena cava.
- D. 3–5 cm of the ascending aorta in the long-axis plane.

113. The propagation speed of sound in a medium is inversely related to the:
- A. elasticity of the media.
- B. temperature of the media.
- C. compressibility of the media.
- D. density of the media.

114. Increasing propagation speed differences will:
- A. decrease the degree of refraction.
- B. produce no change in refraction.
- C. increase attenuation.
- D. increase the refraction angle.

115. The equation for far field divergence is:
- A. $d^2/4$ LAMBDA.
- B. SIN = 1.22 LAMBDA/D.
- C. $d^2/4 \times$ wavelength.
- D. COS = 1.25 LAMBDA/D.

116. Determinants of propagation speed are:
1. elasticity.
2. temperature.
3. permeability.
4. density.
5. contour.
- A. 1, 2, and 3

- B. 1, 2, and 4
- C. 1, 2, and 5
- D. 2 and 4

117. Which of the following is characteristic of axial resolution?
- A. Ability of the imaging system to resolve two interfaces of minimal distance that lie in a plane perpendicular to the ultrasound beam
- B. Increases with increasing pulse duration
- C. Decreases with decreasing pulse duration
- D. Increases with decreasing pulse duration

118. Attenuation with range results from the effects of:
- A. reflection, refraction, scatter, and compressibility.
- B. reflection, scatter, absorption, and demodulation.
- C. refraction, reflection, scatter, and absorption.
- D. reflection, refraction, compression, and absorption.

119. The dynamic range of signal amplitude is typically:
- A. 30–60 dB.
- B. 40–70 dB.
- C. 50–70 dB.
- D. 10–50 dB.

120. Factors that may influence aliasing include:
1. Nyquist imaging limits.
2. pulse repetition frequency.
3. depth.
4. pulse width.
- A. 1 and 3

B. 2 and 4
C. 2, 3, and 4
D. 1, 2, and 3

121. The presence of a large packet size has what effect on color Doppler sensitivity?
A. Increases sensitivity
B. Decreases sensitivity
C. Must be coupled with clutter filter for any Doppler effect
D. No change in sensitivity

122. The embryonic heart develops as a primitive vascular tube within the pericardial space and is composed of:
1. sinus venosus.
2. bulbous cordis.
3. cardiac loop
4. atrial ventricular valves
A. 1, 2, and 3
B. 1 and 2
C. 2 and 4
D. 4

123. Cardiac output is most accurately calculated from:
A. the aorta.
B. mitral valve inflow.
C. tricuspid valve inflow.
D. the pulmonary artery.

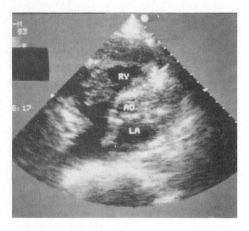

Figure 6-18. Modified short-axis view.

124. The abnormality demonstrated in Figure 6-18 is most consistent with:
A. thrombus.
B. myxoma.
C. vegetation.
D. cardiac neoplasm.

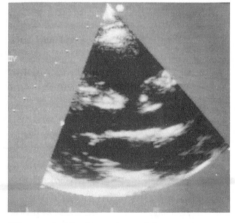

Figure 6-19. Parasternal long-axis view.

125. The image in Figure 6-19 is most consistent with:
A. ventricular septal defect.
B. truncus arteriosus.
C. tetralogy of Fallot.
D. endocardial cushion defect.

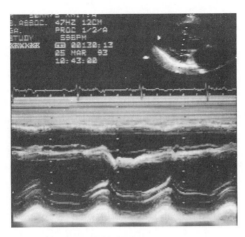

Figure 6-20. M-mode recording distal to the mitral valve.

126. The M-mode tracing in Figure 6-20 is most consistent with:
    A. atrial septal defect.
    B. anteroseptal wall myocardial infarction.
    C. restrictive cardiomyopathy.
    D. constrictive pericarditis.

127. The Doppler tracing in Plate 6-4 corresponds to:
    A. mild mitral valve stenosis.
    B. pericardial effusion.
    C. constrictive pericarditis.
    D. restrictive cardiomyopathy.

128. Two-dimensional criteria for the diagnosis of hypertrophic cardiomyopathy include:
    1. Small- or normal-size left ventricle with normal or hyperdynamic left ventricular function.
    2. hypokinetic intraventricular septum.
    3. asymmetrical septal hypertrophy.
    4. left atrial dilatation.
    A. 1 and 3
    B. 2 and 4
    C. 1, 2, and 3
    D. 4

129. Janeway lesions are signs of:
    A. mitral valve disease.
    B. congenital heart disease.
    C. infective endocarditis.
    D. peripheral vascular disease.

130. Doppler echocardiographic quantification of aortic stenosis is commonly performed from the:
    A. apical view.
    B. parasternal short-axis view.
    C. subcostal view.
    D. low parasternal view.

131. The two-dimensional color-flow Doppler image in Plate 6-5 represents:
    A. atrial septal defect.
    B. pulmonic insufficiency.
    C. patent ductus arteriosis.
    D. aorto-pulmonary artery fistula.

ANSWERS

1. C. The mitral valve consists of two large leaflets and two small commissural cusps. The mitral valve leaflets actually represent a continuous veil of fibrous tissue whose base is attached around the entire circumference of the mitral valve orifice to the fibromuscular ring, the mitral annulus. The anterior leaflet is relatively long and semicircular or triangular, and projects downward into the left ventricular cavity. Although the posterior leaflet is shorter, its attachment to the annulus is more extensive. Among its characteristics, the posterior leaflet of the mitral valve produces a "clapping hands" or paradoxical motion as it moves opposite the anterior leaflet.[6]

2. A. The most consistent echographic finding of mitral stenosis is the reduction of the E-F slope of the anterior leaflet of the valve (velocity of E-F slope measuring less than 35 mm/s). Since the E-F slope is an indicator of the rate of left atrial emptying, in mitral stenosis the decreased slope signifies an obstruction caused by the stenosed orifice. However, it is worth noting that many things other than mitral stenosis may affect the E-F slopes.[6, 11, 23]

3. D. The uppermost part of the right ventricle, the *infundibulum*, has smooth walls without any projecting muscle bundles, and leads into the pulmonary artery.[23]

4. D. Aortic insufficiency (AI) permits the leaking of blood back into the left ventricle during diastole. Regurgitation may be secondary to abnormal aortic cusps or dilatation of the aortic root or ascending aorta. A common cause of chronic AI is rheumatic fever, which causes the cusps to become thickened, fibrotic, and shrunken. Connective tissue diseases such as Marfan's syndrome commonly cause ascending aortic dilatation, as do inflammatory processes such as syphilitic aortitis.[6]

5. C. The aortic valve lies at the root of the aorta and contains three cusps. The wall of the aorta bulges out adjacent to each cusp to form the sinus of Valsalva, sometimes referred to as the *aortic annulus*.[7, 23]

6. D. Mitral valve motion is influenced by many factors, including the relative pressures within the left ventricle and left atrium, the velocity and volume of blood through its orifice, the motion of the leaflets in reference to their annular attachment, the left ventricle diastolic compliance, and the systolic performance of the left ventricle.[6]

7. C. One of the first echographic findings of coronary artery disease

is abnormal wall motion. *Hypokinesis* describes little movement, *hyperkinesis* describes overactive movement, *dyskinesis* describes paradoxical or fragmentary movement, and *akinesis* describes no movement. If interventricular septal motion is abnormal, there is probably a proximal left anterior descending or left main coronary artery obstruction. However, normal septal motion in no way precludes the possibility of partial obstruction in these arteries.[7]

8. B. On phonocardiograms, point C for the mitral valve coincides with the first heart sound, representing the position of maximum closure of the mitral valve.[10]

9. D. The heart is a muscular organ that acts as a double pump: the right side of the heart handles deoxygenated blood, the left side handles oxygenated blood. The human heart is divided longitudinally into right and left halves, each consisting of two chambers: an atrium and a ventricle. The cavities of the atria and ventricles on either side communicate with each other, but the *right and left sides* do not.[23]

10. D. When technical limitations (such as emphysema or an extremely low diaphragm) limit parasternal or apical approaches and preclude gathering of optimal images, the use of subcostal views may significantly increase the chances of deriving clinically useful echocardiographic information.[6]

11. D. The visceral layer (or epicardium) is thin and firmly adherent to the outer heart surface and cannot be easily separated. The visceral layer reflects back on itself at the vascular entry and exit level. This reflection forms the oblique sinus of the pericardium.[6, 23]

12. A. The "swinging heart" motion pattern occurs in large pericardial effusions and frequently suggests the presence of tamponade.[6, 10]

13. D. When ventricular pressure falls below atrial pressure the intake valves open, blood flows into the ventricle, and the filling phase begins.[6, 11, 23]

14. D. Echocardiographic findings in patients with alcoholic cardiomyopathy are similar to those in patients with ischemic cardiomyopathy. Such patients demonstrate increased size of the left ventricular cavity in both systole and diastole, with a decreased ejection fraction. The posterior wall of the left ventricle and the septum tend to be thin, with decreased mobility. Patients exhibit global hypokinesis. Segmental wall motion abnormalities are usually consistent with ischemic cardiomyopathy.[6, 23]

15. D. The left atrium contains the openings of the four pulmonary veins from the lungs.[23]

16. B. Patients with Marfan's syndrome commonly suffer from dilatation of the ascending aorta. They also suffer from aortic insufficiency and may demonstrate dilatation of the pulmonic artery.[6]

17. A. A groove marks the separation between atria and ventricles (the atrioventricular groove or coronary sulcus) in which the right coronary artery lies.[23]

18. D. With ventricular contraction or ventricular systole, the rising pressure in the ventricular cavity closes the atrioventricular valves. As the pressure increases in the ventricles, the semilunar valves (pulmonary and aortic) open so that blood can be forced into the lungs and body, respectively.[6, 10]

19. B. The left ventricle is an egg-shaped structure whose smaller end represents its apex and contains the ventricular outflow tract. The larger end lies at the base of the heart and contains a short inflow tract ranging from the mitral valve to the trabecular zone, and merges with the outflow tract extending to the aortic valve. The anterior leaflet of the mitral valve is continuous with the posterior aortic root, and the interventricular septum is continuous with the anterior aortic root.[10, 23]

20. A. Medial to the tricuspid orifice in the right atrium is the opening for the coronary sinus, which carries blood from the veins of the heart. It is guarded by the coronary, or thebesian, valve.[23]

21. C. The mitral valve opens to a peak at point A by atrial contraction and begins to close after atrial relaxation. Following ventricular contraction, it closes completely at point C. The valve reopens rapidly after the second heart sound and reaches its maximum opening at point E.[6]

22. B. At the cranial end of the conus arteriosus lies the pulmonary orifice with the pulmonary valve. This valve lies cranial and to the left of the tricuspid valve and cranially to the aortic valve.[6]

23. D. The circulatory system and its related organs include the heart and blood vessels (cardiac apparatus), the blood and lymph, lymphatic vessels and related structures, and blood-forming and blood-destroying tissues.[6]

24. B. The pulmonary circulation carries blood from the heart to the lungs via the pulmonary arteries and back to the heart via the pulmonary veins. The pulmonary veins enter the left atrium via four vessels, two from each lung.[23]

25. A. Due to the vibrations of valvular closure, a distinct heart sound is created. The first sound, a low-pitched "lub," is associated with AV valve closure at the beginning of systole.[23]

26. A. The companion of the left coronary artery is the great cardiac vein, which follows the interventricular branch of the artery and the circumflex artery.[23]

27. B. When ejection begins, atrial pressure usually drops sharply, since the atrial floor is pulled down by the contracting ventricles. However, it gradually rises as it receives blood from the veins.[6, 23]

28. C. The heart muscle is autorhythmic (capable of spontaneous, rhythmic self-excitation). Certain cardiac cells, the so-called pacers or pacemakers, have the fastest inherent "firing" rhythm. The primary "pacer" is a small mass of specialized myocardial cells embedded in the right atrial wall near the entrance of the superior vena cava. It is called the sinoatrial (SA) node, and is considered the normal pacemaker for the entire heart.[23]

29. A. A single cardiac cycle is divided into two parts: ventricular contraction (systole) and ventricular relaxation (diastole). The cycle takes about 0.8 seconds from a heart beating at 75 contractions/minute. Systole takes 0.28 seconds, while diastole takes 0.52 seconds. Diastole, therefore, lasts almost twice as long as systole.[23]

30. B. The tricuspid orifice, or atrioventricular opening, is found in the anterior wall of the right atrium and is large enough to admit three fingers.[23]

31. B. The cavity of the left ventricle is longer and narrower than the right, but its walls are much thicker since it has to force blood to the head and body. The papillary muscles are less numerous and stronger, with chordae tendinae from each passing to both cusps of the mitral valve.[23]

32. E
33. C
34. G
35. A

36. F
37. I
38. B
39. H
40. J
41. D[8]

42. B. A prolonged or unusual conduction route in which the impulse always meets an area that is no longer refractory and thus keeps traveling around the heart is a so-called circus movement and may lead to continuous, disorganized contractions, called fibrillation, and even death.[23]

43. B. The cardiovascular system is essentially a closed transport system. It is composed of two major subdivisions: a pulmonary circulation (carrying blood to and from the lungs) and a systemic circulation (carrying blood to all parts of the body and returning it back to the heart).[23]

44. D. As systole begins, a depolarization wave passes through the ventricles and ventricular pressure begins to rise sharply. This immediately closes the AV valves to prevent backflow into the atria, producing the first heart sound which signals the onset of ventricular systole.[6, 10, 23]

45. D. The right pulmonary artery is longer than the left and divides into three primary branches, one for each lobe of the right lung. The left pulmonary artery divides into two primary branches for the two lobes of the left lung.[23]

46. B. Normally, the total volumes of blood pumped through the pulmonary and systemic circuits during a given period of time are equal; that is, the right heart pumps the same amount of blood as the left heart.[23]

47. B. Stimulation of the parasympathetics to the SA node results in a slowing of the heart, and if strong enough, even stops it.[23]

48. C. The aortic opening is surrounded by a fibrous ring to which the bases of the cusps of the aortic semilunar valve are attached. Like the pulmonary semilunar valve, this also has three cusps.[23]

49. A. The chordae tendinae—strong fibrous cords covered with endothelium—extend from the appropriate papillary muscles, attaching to the free edges of the atrioventricular valves and holding them in

place so that they cannot open into the atrium during ventricular systole.[6, 23]

50. B. Near the end of diastole, the SA node fires, the atria depolarize and one sees the "P" wave on an electrocardiogram, and the atria contract.[23]

51. B. With regard to heart valve sounds and their thoracic projection, the pulmonary valve is best heard at the third left costal carti-lage near the sternum (opposite the actual position of the valve proper).[23]

52. A. With hypertrophic cardiomyopathy, typically the size and volume of the left ventricle are normal or reduced. Systolic pressure gradi-ents across the left ventricular outflow tract are common. Charac-teristic morphologic changes (e.g., muscle fiber disarray) are usually most severe in the interventricular septum.[6]

53. B. Ebstein's anomaly is a congenital atrial, ventricular, and tri-cuspid abnormality in which one or more of the tricuspid leaflets are displaced inferiorly into the right ventricular cavity. This mal-formation is usually associated with an atrial septal defect.[6, 10, 23]

54. D[6]

55. B[6]

56. B. Cor triatrium is a congenital anomaly in which a membrane that results from fusion of the common pulmonary veins and the embryonic left atrium does not regress completely. A fibrous mem-brane remains, which divides the left atrium into upper and lower chambers. The membrane is located immediately superior to the left atrial appendage and the fossa ovalis. All of the pulmonary veins drain into the upper chamber. The lower chamber communi-cates with the mitral valve.[6]

57. C. In this parasternal long-axis view, there is evidence of a defect in the anterior leaflet of the mitral valve. Typically, these patients have a deformity of the anterior leaflet with the lateral and medial aspects of the anterior mitral leaflet opened outwardly. The addi-tional abnormality most commonly seen with this type of valve is an ostium primum atrial septal defect. It should be noted that this patient shows evidence of increased echogenicity in the proximal portion of the intraventricular septum related to closure of a ven-tricular septal defect in the past. The patient also had an ostium

primum defect closed. On color-flow Doppler there was evidence of both mitral regurgitation centrally located and a proximal eccentric jet coursing through the anterior leaflet defect.[24]

58. C. An ostium primum atrial septal defect is a common feature in the presence of a cleft mitral valve. This is a form of partial endocardial cushion defect. However, a complete endocardial cushion defect may be seen involving both atrial and ventricular septa. The long-axis view may reveal paradoxical ventricular septal motion if right ventricular volume overload is unopposed, and a narrow goose neck deformity of the left ventricular outflow tract may be present.[24]

59. C. The sinus of Valsalva aneurysm is a rare anomaly that may involve a singular sinus or multiple sinuses. Although the majority of focal aneurysms are congenital, trauma may also precipitate an aneurysm. In this case, the etiology was infective endocarditis. The right coronary sinus is most commonly involved, and the first signs of rupture may be the onset of congestive heart failure. The most common sites of rupture are into the right ventricle and right atrium.[14, 26]

60. B. This multicolored aliased flow disturbance with shunt flow into the right atrium was noted in the region of the right sinus of Valsalva. Color-flow Doppler provides definitive evidence of shunt flow from the sinus into the right atrium, which is a common presentation for this lesion. The presence of the two-dimensional finding coupled with the Doppler findings provides a concrete diagnosis for this abnormality.[14]

61. D. Mitral valve stenosis is characterized by thickened or deformed leaflets, abnormal restrictive diastolic leaflet motion, and reduction in the mitral valve orifice. The characteristic diastolic dome of the mitral valve is noted in this example. This pattern is best recorded in the parasternal long-axis view. Quantitation of this lesion is best assessed with Doppler echocardiography by calculating orifice size from the pressure half-time formula.[6]

62. A. Doppler echocardiography provides the ability to quantitate mitral stenosis through the pressure half-time formula. This formula states that the time required for the peak velocity to be reduced by one-half is quantitatively related to the degree of mitral stenosis. Multiply the peak velocity of the E point by 0.7; the time (m/s) required for the velocity to drop to that particular value is the pressure half-time. This figure is then added into the formula:

$$\text{mitral valve area (MVA)} = \frac{220}{\text{pressure half-time}}$$

[8]

63. D. This M-mode example reveals evidence of akinesis of the posterior lateral wall and increased echogenicity consistent with scarring. Such findings, in which compensatory hyperdynamic septal motion is present and the LV chamber is mildly enlarged, are consistent with a circumflex artery occlusion.[11]

64. C. The presence of papillary muscle dysfunction is common in the presence of posterior wall myocardial infarction. The severity of the mitral valve regurgitation due to papillary muscle dysfunction is variable and depends on fluctuating degrees of ischemia of the papillary muscle or the surrounding myocardium, as well as the systolic blood pressure. Generally, the mitral valve regurgitation is mild; however, in the presence of severe left ventricular dysfunction the mitral valve regurgitation may become a significant factor contributing to congestive heart failure.[12]

65. B. The presence of echogenicity in the left ventricular outflow tract along with a multilayered, shaggy appearance is consistent with vegetation. The prolapsing vegetation attached to the aortic valve allows the mass to enter the left ventricular outflow tract during diastole. The increased M-mode sampling rate provides extremely high resolution documentation of the fine, layered, shaggy-appearing vegetation.[8, 20]

66. A[8, 20]

67. D. Calculating pulmonary artery systolic pressure is accomplished by a continuous-wave recording of the maximal velocity of the tricuspid regurgitation obtained from the apex of the right ventricle. Utilizing $4V^2$ formula, the peak tricuspid pressure drop is calculated in mm/hg. The estimation of right atrial pressure is accomplished by assessing inferior vena cava collapsibility, normal being an inspiratory collapse of greater than 40%. Therefore, pulmonary artery systolic pressure = pressure drop across tricuspid valve + right atrial pressure expressed in mm/hg.[9]

68. D. The rupture of a papillary muscle or a chordae tendinae is detectable by two-dimensional echocardiography. The flail mitral leaflet can usually be distinguished from marked prolapse by the loss of leaflet coaptation during systole, when either the anterior or posterior leaflet moves chaotically back into the left atrium in a systolic flailing motion. Doppler echocardiography usually confirms the presence of severe mitral valve regurgitation.[9]

69. B. The presence of severely enlarged right heart chambers should alert the sonographer to the possibility of atrial septal defect. Os-

tium secundum defect is the most common and suggested in this scan by dropout of this region of the interatrial septum. The left ventricle and left atrium are "pancaked" by the right heart enlargement. Doppler findings of a significant left-to-right shunt would be probable. The best views from which to obtain this information are parasternal short axis, apical four chamber, and subcostal.[19]

70. A. This case represents an example of a constrictive pericardium, and in this instance is evidence of an abnormal notching of the interventricular septum in early diastole, along with evidence of exaggerated left and right ventricular size changes during inspiration and expiration. Additional characteristic signs can be demonstrated with M-mode, two-dimensional, and Doppler echocardiography. A hallmark Doppler feature is demonstration of excessive inspiratory decrease in the mitral E point velocity on the first heart beat after inspiration. The reverse is true of the tricuspid inflow. There may be a dense-appearing pericardium, dilated inferior vena cava, and hepatic veins lacking inspiratory collapse.[3]

71. C. The visceral pericardium, or epicardium, is separated from the parietal pericardium in the presence of a pericardial effusion.[7]

72. B. Right ventricular volume overload, for whatever reason, may cause paradoxical septal motion. The most common reasons for right ventricular overload (either pressure- or volume-related) include an acutely large pulmonary embolism or atrial septal defect with left-to-right shunting, whether it be secundum or primum defect. Other conditions that cause paradoxical motion of the ventricular septum include cardiac surgery, left bundle branch block, absence of the pericardium and Type B Wolf-Parkinson-White syndrome, or severe chronic obstructive pulmonary disease.[9]

73. A. The presence of thinning of the myocardium and increased echogenicity is consistent with scar formation. There is evidence of a significant amount of wall affected by a left anterior descending artery stenosis. Therefore, left ventricular function is compromised, leading to decreased left ventricular ejection fraction and possibly a complication of myocardial infarction—congestive heart failure. Serial echocardiographic studies in this instance may be of significant benefit to follow left ventricular function and possible development of left ventricular aneurysm or thrombus formation.[6]

74. D. The velocity is measured from the baseline to the peak systolic flow. The formula for the peak gradient in millimeters of mercury is $4V^2$, in which gradients greater than 65 mm/hg are considered severe.[6]

75. C. The aortic valve area may be calculated from the continuity equation. From the parasternal long-axis view, the diameter of the left ventricular outflow tract is measured just proximal to the aortic valve. From the apical four-chamber view, the peak left ventricular outflow tract velocity is obtained with pulsed-wave Doppler technique. This sample is taken at the left ventricular outflow tract. The peak velocity is measured across the valve with continuous-wave Doppler. The formula is:

aortic valve area (AVA) in cm
    = LVOT velocity × LVOT area ÷ aortic peak velocity   [6]

76. A[25]

77. B. Mitral valve regurgitation is often observed in patients with myocardial infarction. The causative factors include asynergy of the papillary muscle or ventricular wall that results in mitral valve regurgitation. This may also occur in relation to mitral annular dilatation. The severity of the mitral valve regurgitation due to papillary muscle dysfunction is variable, and depends on the degree of ischemia of the papillary muscles or the surrounding myocardium. It has been demonstrated that papillary muscle infarction does not produce significant mitral valve regurgitation unless both papillary muscles or left ventricular myocardium adjacent to a single infarcted papillary muscle are also involved.[9]

78. C. The presence of a significant area of myocardial damage precipitates symptoms of congestive heart failure including dyspnea precipitated by pulmonary edema or possible peripheral edema related to right ventricular failure. Additionally, if recurrent angina does occur, this would implicate the presence of infarct expansion or possibly a separate, remote lesion in the coronary tree. Rhythm abnormalities are a significant complication of acute myocardial infarction and must be monitored closely in the in-hospital setting. Most deaths among patients with acute myocardial infarction who reach the hospital are attributable to left ventricular failure and subsequent shock, occurring within the first four days of onset of infarction. A reduced amount of in-hospital deaths are now the result of primary arrhythmias. Pre-hospital deaths are primarily related to acute arrhythmias.[4]

79. B. The list of indications for transesophageal echocardiography (TEE) continues to grow. However, there are certain specific conditions in which TEE has been shown to be clinically useful. These include a cardiac source of embolus, prosthetic valve dysfunction, intraoperative trauma and dissection, endocarditis, and complex le-

sions related to congenital heart disease. The sensitivity of TEE technique is superior to transthoracic echocardiographic examination.[18]

80. D. The degree of mitral valve regurgitation is graded according to the size of jet area. Regurgitant severity is graded as follows: an area less than 3 cm is mild, areas of 3 to 6 cm are moderate, and areas of 6 cm or greater are severe. There is agreement with this system of grading and angiographic grading of mitral valve regurgitation. Generally, the surface echocardiographic study underestimates the severity of mitral valve regurgitation, primarily due to the prosthetic valve artifact attenuation and inability to interrogate at an optimum angle with Doppler techniques.[18]

81. C. In the presence of acute aortic valve regurgitation there is evidence of early closure of the mitral valve related to excessive increases in left ventricular pressures exceeding left atrial pressures prior to the onset of mechanical left ventricular systole. Echocardiographic studies have demonstrated that premature closure of the mitral valve is a sensitive and specific indicator for severe aortic insufficiency, and that such early closure is related to the mechanism of Austin-Flynt murmur.[9]

82. B. An infiltrative cardiomyopathy is characterized by thickened myocardium ("ground glass, mottled appearance"), multiple valvular thickenings with regurgitation, poor left ventricular function, and pericardial effusion. Prognosis is poor. Amyloidosis is the most common type of known infiltrative cardiomyopathy.[6]

83. C. There is color-flow Doppler evidence of a high velocity jet entering from the posterior aortic root into the left atrium. This is consistent with an aortic left atrial fistula related to endocarditis. This presentation is quite dramatic and can be progressive with precipitation of congestive heart failure by expansion of the fistula into the adjacent cardiac chamber. The beauty of the Doppler color mapping allows simultaneous visualization of the blood-flow signal superimposed on the two-dimensional image. This patient was later taken to surgery for repair of the aortic valve and fistula with good results.[13]

84. D. The presence of a significant pericardial effusion precipitates increased inferior vena cava dimension with poor collapse on inspiration, evidence of right atrial collapse, or right ventricular early diastolic collapse as well as marked variation (more than 30 percent during respiration) in Doppler transvalvular flow velocity. In addition, a marked variation in ventricular size is noted during the respiratory cycle, that is, inspiratory increase in the right ventricular

dimension and decreases in the left ventricular dimension. The mitral valve may show rather bizarre motion as the heart swings consistent with pseudo-anterior motion of the mitral valve. Paradoxical motion of the interventricular septum is related to significant alterations in ventricular pressure and volume and is dependent on the amount of pericardial effusion.[15]

85. A. Cardiac metastasis occurs with all types of primary tumors, carcinomas, sarcomas, leukemias, lymphomas, and melanomas. No malignant tumor tends to particularly metastasize to the heart, with the possible exception of malignant melanoma, which involves the myocardium in over 50 percent of cases.[12]

86. D. Almost all primary malignant cardiac tumors are sarcomas, most frequently angiosarcomas. They originate in the right atrium or pericardium. One-fourth of all angiosarcomas will in part be intracavitary with valvular obstruction. They may manifest with right-sided failure and pericardial tamponade with bloody fluid. The prognosis is poor with rapid, widespread metastases.[12]

87. C. Cardiac thrombi may be observed in the left ventricle and the left atrium. In the presence of a patent foramen ovale (PFO) or atrial septal defect (ASD), a potential pathway exists for paradoxical embolization. Transesophageal echocardiography is superior in identifying left atrial appendage thrombus PFOs and small ASDs in comparison to transthoracic examination. It is well known that patients with atrial fibrillation and left atrial enlargement have a high incidence of left atrial thrombus formation. In addition, several investigators have shown that left atrial thrombus may be identified in individuals in sinus rhythm with no detectable morphologic or functional cardiac disease. Left ventricular thrombus identification ranges from 80% to 90% with transthoracic examination. This is the result of the superior apical windows usually obtained with transthoracic approaches.[18]

88. C. Characteristics of hypertrophic cardiomyopathy include asymmetrical septal hypertrophy, narrow left ventricular outflow tract, and high position of the mitral valve apparatus with the interventricular septum in systole. The septal myocardium may appear to be more echo-reflectant, presumably due to abnormally arranged myocardial cells. The left ventricular dimension is usually small with encroachment on the hypertrophied walls. If there is an obstruction present, the characteristic systolic anterior motion of the mitral valve apparatus is appreciated. The mitral valve may be distorted—particularly that of the posterior leaflet, which appears to be

elongated—the coaptation point being at a more basal portion of the leaflet instead of the leaflet edges. This condition may produce residual leaflet tissue that is drawn toward the intraventricular septum during systole. Left atrial enlargement may also be noted secondary to the presence of mitral valve regurgitation and chronic elevation of left ventricular filling pressures.[11]

89. B. M-mode findings of hypertrophic cardiomyopathy are very similar to that of two-dimensional exams. Better resolution does, however, provide additional findings of mid-systolic closure of the aortic valve, more sensitive identification of systolic anterior motion of the mitral valve, and possibly more accurate measurement of left ventricular wall thickness. A ratio of the septum to posterior wall thickness of greater than 1.3:1 is consistent with asymmetrical septal hypertrophy (ASH).[11]

90. B. The origin of the second heart sound is attributed to the closure of the semilunar valves, the aortic and pulmonary valves. Because the aortic valve closes before the pulmonary valve, the second heart sound is typically split into two components. Respiration allows a variation in the interval between the aortic and pulmonary components. The components split during inspiration and merge during expiration in most normal persons.[28]

91. B. The echocardiographic findings on M-mode examination usually reveal left and right ventricular enlargement with an abnormal indices of left ventricular function. This would include decreased ejection fraction and fractional shortening. The amplitude of separation of the mitral valve leaflets is decreased and the mitral apparatus may be located posteriorly. Miniaturization of the mitral valve may be present, related to decreased cardiac output and decreased volumes flowing through the mitral valve during cardiac output and decreased volumes flowing through the mitral valve during diastole. Abnormal closure of the mitral valve, as noted by a B-notch, signifies elevated left ventricular end diastolic filling pressures. A pericardial effusion is commonly seen and mural thrombi may be found. The two-dimensional examination provides increased sensitivity in identifying mural thrombi and evaluating for segmental wall-motion abnormalities in patients with an underlying ischemic cardiomyopathy.[6]

92. C. Three major coronary arteries and their tributaries supply the myocardium: the right coronary artery, the left anterior descending coronary artery, and the circumflex coronary artery. In Figure 6-16 there is evidence of septal thinning and akinesis consistent with

myocardial infarction. The coronary artery that supplies the anterior wall of the myocardium is the left anterior descending coronary artery. A wall-motion abnormality occurring in the distribution of the left anterior descending artery may involve the septum, anterior wall, and the apex of the left ventricle.[6]

93. C. Although inflow patterns and their characteristic changes in disease are often essential in a clinical diagnosis, one must realize that these patterns are dynamic. Pseudo-normalization may occur if alterations in loading conditions, such as medical therapy or anatomy, mask the changes in the patterns of delayed relaxation of restrictive physiology. Appleton and co-workers have described three dynamic types of mitral velocity filling patterns. They emphasize that the pattern seen in a single patient may shift depending on loading conditions or serial changes in a disease state. In the presence of impaired relaxation, there is a decrease in the E-wave magnitude and an increase in the A-wave, while deceleration time and the isovolumic relaxation time are prolonged. The intermediate pattern is of normal inflow or perhaps pseudo-normalization. This pattern suggests that even though the left ventricular inflow appears normal, there are significant abnormalities of diastolic function. The final pattern is a restrictive pattern with an increased E-wave, a decrease in A-wave amplitude, and a shortened deceleration time with a normal or shortened isovolumic relaxation time. Therefore, by changing preload in a patient with an abnormal relaxation pattern, the flow may change completely. Patients with delayed left ventricular relaxation who develop an increase in left atrial pressure may pseudo-normalize.[1]

94. F
95. D
96. C
97. A
98. E
99. B

100. D[27]

101. C
102. A
103. D
104. B
105. F
106. E

107. A[25,27]

108. D. Patients with significant mitral valve regurgitation have blunted or reversed pulmonary venous flow. This can be best observed with transesophageal echocardiography, although transthoracic interrogation of the pulmonary veins is also possible. Patients with this pattern usually have moderate to severe mitral valve regurgitation.[5]

109. C. This pattern is representative of a restrictive diastolic filling pattern in which the isovolumic relaxation time (IVRT) is decreased secondary to increased left atrial pressure. In addition, the deceleration time of the mitral valve in early diastole is shortened secondary to the majority of diastolic flow occurring in early diastole. This pattern is seen in the presence of restrictive cardiomyopathy, such as cardiac amyloidosis, usually in the latter stages of this disease. It should be noted that restrictive patterns of this type correlate with generally poor prognoses. This pattern can also be seen in the presence of myocardial infarction and dilated cardiomyopathy, in which there is an incidence of higher filling pressures and symptoms of congestive heart failure.[2, 16]

110. D. The examination is consistent with marked increased reversal of flow during inspiration. In addition, there is an increased peak diastolic-to-systolic flow during all phases of respiration. This is in comparison to constrictive pericarditis, where there is a normal increase in peak systolic and diastolic flow velocities during inspiration. However, in expiration, systolic flow velocity decreases and diastolic flow velocity decreases, reflecting decreased flow velocities in the right ventricular inflow. There is also marked increased reversal of flow in the hepatic vein during expiration, consistent with decreases in right ventricular inflow velocities.[16]

111. C. A mitral regurgitant jet area of less than 3 cm seen on transesophageal echocardiography is considered mild mitral valve regurgitation. From 3 to 6 cm is moderate mitral valve regurgitation, and a greater than 6-cm area is consistent with severe mitral valve regurgitation. This scale corresponds accurately to angiographic grading of mitral valve regurgitation. In the presence of markedly eccentric jets, which may be seen in patients with a flail mitral valve leaflet, a smaller regurgitant jet area may be present. In these instances, evaluation of the pulmonary venous flow may add additional information in assessing the degree of mitral regurgitation in such patients.[18]

112. C. In the vertical or longitudinal plane, extreme clockwise rotation of the transducer will allow visualization of the right atrium, superior vena cava, and inferior vena cava. Other standard views ob-

tained with longitudinal scanning include two-chamber views of the left atrium and left ventricle, short-axis view of the aorta with the right ventricular inflow and outflow tract, and a long-axis view of the ascending aorta visualizing the first 3 to 5 cm of the vessel.[18]

113. D. Determinants of propagation speed in soft tissues are stiffness, density, compressibility, and temperature. The propagation speed of sound increases as the density of the media decreases. Additionally, propagation speed is directly related to temperature, elasticity, and compressibility.[17]

114. D. Refraction occurs when an incident sound beam that is oblique to an interface changes direction on the transmission side of the interface due to the differences in propagation speeds of the two media. Therefore, increasing the propagation speed differences will increase the degree of refraction or bending of the sound beam. The refraction equation is:

$$\frac{\text{sine of i}}{\text{sine of r}} = \frac{C1}{C2} \qquad [17]$$

115. B. There are two ultrasonic field characteristics: near field and far field, also known as the Fresnel and Fraunhofer zones. The near field offers the best ultrasonic resolution because the sound beam does not undergo divergence. In the far field, beam divergence adversely affects lateral resolution.[17]

116. B. Determinants of propagation speed are elasticity, density, temperature, and compressibility. Propagation (average) speed in soft tissue is 1540 m/s.[17]

117. D. Axial resolution is defined as the ability of the imaging system to resolve two or more interfaces of minimal distance that lie in a plane parallel to the ultrasound beam. Pulse duration is that length of time required to complete one pulse. Therefore, decreasing the pulse duration shortens the length of time required to complete one pulse, allowing more information to be processed. This, in turn, improves axial resolution. Axial resolution is also dependent on spatial pulse length, damping, transducer frequency, and bandwidths.[17]

118. C. The intensity of an ultrasound beam decreases with increasing distance due to the effects of reflection, refraction, scatter, and absorption. The receiver sweep gains or TGC compensates for this loss in amplitude of detected echoes from distant interfacing, as related to normal attenuation of sound in an acoustic media.[17]

119. B. Dynamic range is the range of signal amplitudes from smallest to largest that can be detected and processed by an ultrasound system. The typical dynamic range is from 40 to 70 dB.[17]

120. D. Pulse repetition frequency (PRF), Nyquist frequency limit, and depth baseline position all affect signal ambiguity or aliasing. Aliasing increases with increasing transducer frequency. The Nyquist frequency limit is the PRF divided by 2. The Nyquist frequency may be unusually low with increased transducer frequency, and it is frequently necessary to decrease transducer frequency to prevent aliasing. The farther away the echo target is the more likely aliasing will occur, related to PRF decrease and Nyquist limit decrease.[17]

121. A. The presence of a larger packet size increases the number and timing of ultrasonic bursts per scan line; therefore, with a larger packet size more information is obtained. With color-flow Doppler, a sampling of 6 to 8 packets are used to generate multiple sample gates along each scan line.[17]

122. A. The composition of the primitive heart tube includes the sinus venosus, cardiac loop, and bulbus chordus or the truncus arteriosus. At approximately 4 weeks' gestation, the tube rotates to form the atria and ventricles and the truncus arteriosus. At this time unidirectional blood flow is initiated through the primitive tube. The sinus venosus develops from the umbilical and the vitelline veins. The right and left sinus horns, respectively, develop from the veins as independent chambers. The left horn becomes a coronary sinus and the right horn forms the vena cava. As the tube rotates from the cardiac loop, a primitive single atria and ventricle develop.[21]

123. A. In adults, the most accurate cardiac outputs are obtained from the left ventricular outflow tract or aorta. Values needed to calculate the cardiac output are flow velocity interval (FVI), cross-sectional area (CSA), and heart rate. The Doppler spectral tracing should clearly show the onset and end of flow, a narrow bandwidth, and consistent peak velocities from beat to beat. For the most accurate results, several complexes should be averaged. The cross-sectional area is measured from leading-edge to leading-edge with clear borders visible. An area of 1 to 2 mm is significantly magnified by the formula because of the squaring of the radius. Therefore, stroke volume would equal the FVI times the CSA. This, multiplied by the heart rate, equals cardiac output. Normal cardiac output ranges from 4 to 6 liters per minute.[6]

124. D. Metastatic cardiac tumors are 16 to 40 times more common than primary cardiac tumors. Carcinomatous invasion is more frequent than sarcoma invasion. Cardiac infiltration is seen in over $1/2$ of leukemia cases and in $1/6$ of lymphoma cases (particularly reticulum cell sarcoma). Extensive myocardial infiltration is usually present, and occasionally a major coronary vessel may be occluded. In patients with lymphoma the cardiovascular abnormalities may be due to mediastinal or pulmonary lymphoma, anemia, hypoalbumen, and unrelated cardiac disease. Myxomas are uncommon, accounting for less than 0.5% of all tumors; however, they are considered to be one of the most common cardiac tumors. Myxomas usually occur as pedunculated (arising from a stalk) tumors most commonly attached to the interatrial septum. Although generally benign, when left untreated myxomas can cause death from heart failure, systemic emboli, or valvular dysfunction.[12]

125. C. Tetralogy of Fallot has four dominant components: (1) a moderate to large ventricular septal defect, (2) override of the aorta, (3) obstruction to pulmonary blood flow at any level, and (4) right ventricular hypertrophy. Occasionally, tetralogy of Fallot is discovered in later life if the obstruction is not severe and in patients who have not received regular medical care. These so-called "pink tets" may be able to pursue a normally active life-style until obstruction progresses further. Multiple two-dimensional echo approaches as well as complimentary Doppler investigation are required to assess the types and severity of obstruction seen in these patients.[6]

126. D. M-mode echocardiographic features include pericardial thickening, increased depth of the "a" wave on the pulmonary valve, rapid early and flat mid-diastolic motion of the posterior left ventricle, rapid early and flat mid-diastolic motion of the posterior aortic root, posterior atrial systolic notch on the septum, abnormal early diastolic ventricular septal motion, abrupt anterior or posterior motion, and abnormal septal motion in systole. In the presence of constrictive pericarditis, diastolic expansion is restricted because of the rigid pericardium, and right-sided diastolic pressures are elevated and equal to left-sided diastolic pressures. These elevated right-sided diastolic pressures are equal to or within 5 mm of the left-sided fill in pressures. The presence of early diastolic notching may be related to the early diastolic right-to-left gradient, resulting in a posterior motion of the intraventricular septum early in diastole. The overall clinical significance of constrictive pericarditis is a lowered cardiac output with lowered systemic blood pressures and early fatiguability, as well as peripheral edema and increased dyspnea.[3]

127. C. Constrictive pericarditis involves a thickened nonelastic pericardium. This causes alteration of ventricular filling during inspiration. There is a decrease in mitral valve inflow as noted in Plate 6-4. The reverse occurs in tricuspid valve inflow.[16]

128. C. Hypertrophic cardiomyopathy presents with asymmetrical septal hypertrophy, although concentric LVH has been noted. The septal myocardium may appear more echo-reflectant. If an obstruction is present, the characteristic systolic anterior motion of the mitral valve apparatus can be appreciated. It has also been noted that the posterior leaflet of the mitral valve may be involved with the abnormal anterior motion. Hemodynamically, the abnormal mitral valve motion results in a mid-systolic cessation of blood flow and a partial closure of the aortic valve. During this time, mitral valve regurgitation may be seen. Clinically, these patients present with dyspnea on exertion and presyncope or syncope related to cardiac arrhythmias. Transient ischemic episodes may also occur.[6]

129. C. Janeway lesions are flat, nontender red spots that are small in size (less than 5 mm) and irregular in outline. They are found on the palms and soles of some patients with subacute bacterial endocarditis and acute bacterial endocarditis. Unlike petechiae, they are not hemorrhagic and therefore will blanch on pressure. Additional physical findings in patients with endocarditis include splinter hemorrhages (which occur in approximately 10% of patients), Oslar's nodes (10–20% of patients), eye lesions, embolization, and splenomegaly. The presence of fever, edema, and murmur should suggest endocarditis.[12]

130. A. The apical position would be best. Excellent correlations between Doppler and basic hemodynamics have been widely published. To achieve these results, an experienced imager should interrogate from multiple windows to obtain the highest peak velocities. In the presence of atrial fibrillation, serial measurements of the left ventricular outflow tract and averaging several cardiac cycles should be obtained.[22]

131. C. This color-flow Doppler examination reveals evidence of reverse flow in the region of the pulmonary artery; this is documented as a red-shaded color-flow jet in Plate 6-5 (parasternal short-axis view). The most common type of systemic to pulmonary shunt is a patent ductus arteriosus (PDA). Others include aortic to pulmonary artery window and surgically created shunts. Reversal of flow in the descending aorta may be due to severe aortic regurgitation and insufficiency. In preterm infants, PDA is often closed successfully with the administration of Indomethacin. However, Indomethacin is inef-

fective in the treatment of term infants. PDAs may be corrected by interventional catheterization or surgery. Interventional catheterization techniques involve catheter placement of a foam plastic plug or an umbrella device within the ductus to occlude the lumen. Surgical correction involves ligation with transection. PDAs at times may be desirable, as in the case of complex congenital heart disease in which the ductus may be necessary to maintain communication between the pulmonary and systemic circulation. In such cases, prostaglandin E_1 is administered until a pulmonary systemic shunt can be surgically created.[6]

REFERENCES

1. Appleton CP, Hatle LK, Popp RL. Relation of transmitral flow velocity patterns to left ventricular diastolic functions: new insights from a combined hemodynamic and Doppler echocardiographic study. J Am Coll Cardiol II 1988;12:426.

2. Appleton CP, Hatle LK, Popp RL. Natural history of left ventricular filling abnormalities. Echocardiography 1992;6(4):437.

3. Bansal RC, Chandrasekaran K. Role of echocardiography and Doppler techniques in the evaluation of pericardial diseases. Echocardiography 1989;6(4):293.

4. Braunwald E, ed. Heart disease: a textbook of cardiovascular medicine. 3rd ed. Philadelphia: Harcourt Brace Jovanovich, 1988.

5. Castello R, Pearson AC, Lenzen P, Labovitz AJ. Effect of mitral regurgitation on pulmonary venous velocities derives from transesophageal echocardiography, color guided pulse Doppler. J Am Coll Cardiol 1991;17(7):1499.

6. Craig M. Diagnostic medical sonography. Vol II: Echocardiography. Philadelphia: JB Lippincott, 1991.

7. Dorland's illustrated medical dictionary. 25th ed. Philadelphia: WB Saunders, 1974.

8. Feigenbaum H. Echocardiography. Philadelphia: Lea & Febiger, 1986.

9. Hagan AD, Demaria AW. Clinical applications of two-dimensional echocardiography and cardiac Doppler. Boston: Little Brown, 1989.

10. Hagen-Ansert SL. Textbook of diagnostic ultrasonography. 2nd ed. St. Louis: CV Mosby, 1983.

11. Harrigan P, Lee R. Principles of interpretation in echocardiography. New York: Wiley Medical, 1985.

12. Hirst JW, ed. The heart, arteries, and veins. New York: McGraw-Hill, 1982.

13. Jain SP, Mahan EF, Nanda NC. Doppler color-flow mapping in the diagnosis of sinus of Valsalva aneurysm. Echocardiography 1989;6(6):533.

14. Katz ES, Cziner DG, Rosenzweig BP, et al. Multifaceted echocardiographic approach to the diagnosis of a ruptured sinus of Valsalva aneurysm. Am Soc Echocardiog J III 1991;5:494.

15. King WS, Pandain NG, Gardin JM. Doppler echocardiographic findings in pericardial tamponade and constriction. Echocardiography 1988;5(5):361.

16. Klein AL, Cohen GI. Doppler echocardiographic assessment of constrictive pericarditis, cardiac amyloidosis and cardiac tamponade. Cleveland Clin J Med 1992;59:278.

17. Kremkau FW. Diagnostic ultrasound: principles, instruments and exercises. Philadelphia: WB Saunders, 1989.

18. Labovitz AJ, Pearson AC. Transesophageal echocardiography: basic principles and clinical applications. Philadelphia: Lea & Febiger, 1993.

19. Lin FC, Morgan F, San-Jou Y, et al. Doppler atrial shunt flow pattern in patients with secundum atrial septal defect. J Am Soc Echocardiog 1988;1(3):141.

20. McLeod K, DeLange M, Racker H. Echocardiography of atrial myxomas. J Diag Med Sonog 1990;6(1):19.

21. Netter FH. Ciba collection of medical illustrations. Vol V: The heart. Rochester, NY: Case-Hoyt Corp, 1978.

22. Otto CM, Pearlman AF, Komess KA. Determination of the stenotic valve area in adults using Doppler echocardiography. J Am Coll Cardiol 1986;7:509.

23. Pansky B. Dynamic anatomy and physiology. New York: Macmillan, 1975.

24. Perloff JK. Clinical recognition of congenital heart disease. Philadelphia: WB Saunders, 1987.

25. Perry CJ, Helmeke F, Nanda NC, et al. Evaluation of aortic insufficiency by Doppler color-flow imagery. J Am Coll Cardiol 1983;9:952.

26. Reynolds T. Pocket handbook of echocardiography. Tucson: Arizona Heart Institute, 1993.

27. Robert E, Klower A. The guide to cardiology. New York: Wiley Medical, 1984.

28. Tavell ME. Clinical phonocardiography and external pulse recording. Chicago: Yearbook Medical Publishers, 1977.

Marveen Craig: *Ultrasound Exam Review*, © 1994 J. B. Lippincott Co.

7

DENISE LEVY

Vascular

OBJECTIVES

Within a relatively short time Doppler ultrasound has been established as a valuable adjunct to arteriographic and other diagnostic efforts through its noninvasive demonstration of the major components of the vascular system. The vascular sonographer must be capable of performing skillful, careful examinations and possess a thorough knowledge of the characteristic normal and abnormal patient responses. In addition, sonographers must often determine if further investigations are needed. Study of the vascular section should reinforce the knowledge acquired by students and novice sonographers, spotlighting their strengths and weaknesses in their examination preparations.

QUESTIONS

Directions

Each of the questions or incomplete statements is followed by several answers or completions. Select the best answer(s) in each case. In the matching sections, answers should be used only once, unless otherwise stated.

1. Doppler frequency shifts fall within the audible range of:
   A. 200 Hz–15 kHz.
   B. 500 Hz–15 kHz.
   C. 500 Hz–50 kHz.
   D. 200 Hz–30 kHz.

2. The color priority control:
   A. determines whether gray scale or color Doppler information will be emphasized.
   B. governs color saturation.
   C. can act as a filter.
   D. all of the above.

3. The intramuscular interval on the middle and lower third of the thigh, which contains the superficial femoral vessels and saphenous nerve, is known as:
   A. the adductor canal.
   B. Cloquet's canal.
   C. Hunter's canal.
   D. A and C

4. The largest Doppler shift is demonstrated by spectral analysis when the ultrasound beam insonates the vessel at a:
   A. 90 degree angle.
   B. 45 degree angle.
   C. 0 degree angle.
   D. 15 degree angle.

5. Which of the following anatomical statements concerning the common carotid artery (CCA) are *untrue*?
   A. The right CCA originates off the innominate artery
   B. Bifurcates at the level of the thyroid cartilage
   C. The left CCA originates off the aortic arch
   D. The internal carotid artery tends to be larger than the external carotid

6. The number of cycles per color line is often referred to as:
   A. packet size.
   B. dwell time.
   C. ensemble length.
   D. all of the above

7. Select the *false* statement from the following list.
   A. Pulsed wave (PW) Doppler has excellent signal-to-noise ratios
   B. PW Doppler may reach SPTs of 1 W/cm^2
   C. PW Doppler examines in a limited frequency range
   D. PW Doppler uses operator-set Doppler angle correction

8. Patients at highest risk for developing atherosclerotic disease are:
   A. cigarette smokers.
   B. leukemics.
   C. diabetics.
   D. A and C

9. Peripheral vascular scanning of the superficial femoral vein

must follow the course of the vessel along the _____ of the thigh and at its inferior aspect, just superior to the knee.
A. outer curve
B. inner curve or "in seam"
C. lateral aspect
D. A and C

10. With color imaging, spectral broadening may be viewed as a "variance." One color is arbitrarily chosen to display the highest range of velocities present. This color is often:
A. yellow.
B. green.
C. red.
D. blue.

11. The Doppler characteristics of malignant ovarian lesions *do not* include:
A. central areas of abnormal vasculature.
B. absence of a diastolic notch.
C. high impedance.
D. low impedance.

12. Prevention of the back flow of blood is achieved by vascular valves. Such valves are commonly seen in the:
A. popliteal veins.
B. great and small saphenous veins.
C. common femoral vein and superficial femoral vein.
D. all of the above

13. Intermittent claudication is the most common presenting symptom in mild-to-moderate atherosclerotic vascular disease. Which of the following is (are) common patient complaints:
A. Joint pain
B. Exercise-related calf, thigh, or buttock pain
C. Resting symptoms of continued burning or nagging lower leg pain
D. Constant leg cramping

14. All of the following statements about abdominal Doppler are true *except*:
A. abdominal arterial flow has a fairly low resistance.
B. abdominal masses produce a spectral appearance of higher systolic peaks and more pronounced diastolic components.
C. arterial flow pulsates with the cardiac cycle.
D. the spectral appearance of abdominal masses is one of low systolic peaks and pronounced diastolic components.

15. The carotid arteries lie:
A. medial to the thyroid gland.
B. lateral to the internal jugular vein.
C. posteromedial to the sternocleidomastoid muscle.
D. posterior and lateral to the esophagus.

16. The _____ mode of Doppler ultrasound is the most sensitive in detecting areas of vascular flow in breast tumors.
A. continuous-wave
B. pulsed-wave

C. color-flow
D. water-path

17. Hepatic arteries tend to demonstrate:
    A. low-impedance flow.
    B. high-impedance flow.
    C. increased postprandial turbulence.
    D. persistently decreasing diastolic flow.

18. False-positive diagnosis of occlusion can result from:
    A. vessel tortuosity.
    B. the presence of plaque.
    C. confusion of the external for the internal carotid artery.
    D. all of the above

19. Spectral analysis employs the use of _____ shades to represent the power or intensity of the Doppler signal.
    A. yellow
    B. blue
    C. gray
    D. green

20. When performing segmental limb pressures, a drop in pressure of _____ mm/hg between segments is an indication of occlusive peripheral vascular disease (PVD) in the intervening segment.
    A. 10–15
    B. 15–20
    C. 20–30
    D. 30–40

21. For a multicuff lower-extremity arterial segment:
    A. four cuffs should be placed on each leg (two above the knee and two below).
    B. three cuffs should be placed on each leg (two above the knee, one below the knee at the calf).
    C. two cuffs should be placed on each leg (one above the knee and one below the knee at the calf).
    D. A and B

22. Color Doppler imaging of the region of Hunter's canal is often difficult because of:
    A. vessel depth.
    B. vessel tortuosity.
    C. excessive collagen deposition.
    D. excessive muscularity.

23. Which of the following is(are) *not* characteristic of chronic DVT (deep vein thrombosis)?
    A. Fresh thrombus may be hypoechoic
    B. Chronic thrombus appears echogenic within 1–2 weeks
    C. Thrombi age has no bearing on compressibility
    D. B and C

24. Colors used for display of color Doppler analyses use:
    A. hue and luminosity.
    B. shades of orange and yellow.
    C. saturation.
    D. A and C

25. Which of the following statements about photoplethysmography are *untrue*?

A. The transducer is applied directly to the toes
B. Relative perfusion of a study area is documented
C. Cutaneous flow is detected
D. None of the above

26. In patients with venous hypertension, abdominal Doppler studies will demonstrate dilation of the splanchnic vessels greater than _____ diameter.
    A. 5 mm
    B. 10 mm
    C. 1.5 cm
    D. .5 cm

Match the following terms to numbers 27–31.

A. Arteriovenous malformations
B. Stenotic grafts
C. Hematomas
D. Pseudoaneurysms
E. "target" appearance

27. ____ A nonvascular hypoechoic mass

28. ____ Two-fold increase in flow velocity

29. ____ Benign nodes

30. ____ Swirling, alternating color patterns of red/blue flow

31. ____ Accentuated venous outflow with arterialized spectral patterns

32. The CW duplex imaging transducer of choice for peripheral vascular scans of the lower extremities is:

A. 3.5–5.0 MHz.
B. 5.0–7 MHz.
C. 10–20 MHz.
D. 1.5–3 MHz.

33. Select the *false* statement concerning abdominal Doppler ultrasound.
    A. The Doppler shift frequency usually falls within the audible frequency range
    B. Doppler shift frequencies increase as operating frequencies increase
    C. The Doppler angle should be set between 60–90 degrees
    D. When examining large vessels, the cursor size should be kept smaller

34. Select the *incorrect* choice from the following statements regarding biological effects.
    A. No known bioeffects have been proved below 100 mW/cm^2 SPTA
    B. Scanning should be carried out only on a "when needed" basis
    C. Fetal heart and umbilical cord Doppler examinations are not approved
    D. Sonographers should scan conscientiously at all times.

35. The lower leg pressures are divided by the arm pressure for an ankle-brachial index (ABI). The normal resting index should be
    A. 1.00–1.39 mm/hg.
    B. 0.91–0.99 mm/hg.
    C. 0.90–1.00 mm/hg.
    D. 0.89–0.98 mm/hg.

36. The presence of biphasic signals in the portal vein suggests:
    A. IVC thrombosis.
    B. portal vein stenosis.
    C. portal vein hypertension.
    D. respiratory variation.

37. Normal posterior tibial artery Doppler signals should be:
    A. monophasic.
    B. biphasic.
    C. triphasic.
    D. quadraphasic.

38. When sampling blood flow, the highest (peak) velocities are most likely to be encountered at:
    A. the widest vessel diameter.
    B. the narrowest vessel diameter.
    C. midvessel.
    D. the site of anastomosis.

39. Color and spectral Doppler examination of the venous patterns in the legs should focus on:
    A. vein compressibility.
    B. presence or absence of intraluminal masses.
    C. signal intensity at rest and with augmentation.
    D. all of the above

40. The color Doppler appearance of aliasing may be recognized as:
    A. the velocities exceed the PRF of the transducer.
    B. abrupt color change caused by flow reversal.
    C. abrupt color change unrelated to flow reversal.
    D. A and C

41. The characteristic resistance of the renal arteries is:
    A. <100 cm/s.
    B. <200 cm/s.
    C. <300 cm/s.
    D. <400 cm/s.

42. Acute vascular rejection is usually not seen in renal transplants until after the _____ week following surgery.
    A. first   C. third
    B. second   D. fourth

43. With the *absence* of lower extremity atherosclerotic disease, postexercise ABI, when compared to preexercise ABI, should demonstrate:
    A. elevation of ankle and brachial pressures.
    B. stable ankle-brachial indexes (ABI).
    C. a drop in ankle pressure and elevated ABIs.
    D. A and B

44. All of the following statements about lower leg venous competence are true *except:*
    A. any flow visible to the transducer with proximal compression represents incompetent valves.
    B. pulsatile venous flow suggests congestive heart failure, fluid overload, or tricuspid insufficiency.
    C. sampling at a point inferior to a valve, when leg compression is exerted superior to the valve, should not result in backflow.
    D. Valsalva maneuvers are ineffective in demonstrating valvular competence.

45. Abnormal plethysmographic signals will *not* demonstrate:
    A. broadening.
    B. decreased amplitude.
    C. attenuation of the dicrotic notch.
    D. loss of the dicrotic notch.

46. The infraorbital artery is a distal branch of the:
    A. temporal artery.
    B. maxillary artery.
    C. transverse facial artery.
    D. superficial temporal artery.

47. Select the *false* statement about Doppler evaluation of breast tumor vascularity.
    A. Reasonably specific for malignancy
    B. May serve as a marker for tumor aggressiveness
    C. Particularly sensitive to malignancy
    D. Is a slow and tedious examination

48. If the Doppler angle is set perpendicular to flow, the computer will be unable to:
    A. detect any reverse flow.
    B. detect forward from reverse flow.
    C. detect any Doppler shift.
    D. detect vessel wall vibrations.

49. Grating lobes occur because:
    A. the sound beam is perpendicular to the target.
    B. the sound beam is not perpendicular to the target.
    C. the transducer frequency is too low.
    D. the system gain is too high.

50. Veins are thin-walled structures composed of _____ tissue layers.
    A. 1
    B. 2
    C. 3
    D. 4

51. The presence of mosaic patterns represents:
    A. low velocity.
    B. high velocity.
    C. complex flow.
    D. B and C

52. Which of the following actions will correct range ambiguity artifacts?
    A. Increasing gain and pulse repetition frequency (PRF)
    B. Decreasing far gain and PRF
    C. Increasing PRF and decreasing far gain
    D. Increasing transducer frequency and far gain

Match the following terms to numbers 53–57.

    A. Augmentation
    B. Claudication
    C. Demodulation
    D. Ischemia
    E. Phasicity

53. ____ Cramping with exercise
54. ____ Quadrature phase detector
55. ____ Compression techniques
56. ____ Respiratory flow variations
57. ____ Localized diminution of arterial blood flow

58. Which of the following statements concerning color Doppler systems is *untrue?*

A. Tend to have poorer resolution
B. Are unable to detect flow less than 1 cm/s
C. Use frame rates of 4–32 frames/s
D. A and C

59. In patients with cellulitis, it is often difficult to visualize the deep leg veins because of:
A. interstitial inflammation.
B. increased echogenicity.
C. increased transmission through fluid.
D. A and B

60. Scrotal Doppler evidence of varicocele includes:
A. venous dilatation of >3 mm during Valsalva maneuver.
B. complete or near complete absence of flow.
C. hypervascularity.
D. high arterial flow.

61. Vascular ulcerations often produce irregularities along the borders of:
A. vessel walls.
B. plaque.
C. thrombus.
D. the intima.

62. The Doppler characteristic(s) of renal transplant rejection is(are):
A. decreasing diastolic flow.
B. increasing capillary resistance.
C. decreasing blood flow.
D. all of the above

63. The use of color Doppler techniques in gynecology includes all of the following *except:*

A. documenting ovulatory flow.
B. documenting ectopic trophoblastic flow.
C. documenting increased flow during follicular ovulation phases.
D. documenting increased peak systolic flow in active ovaries.

64. The patient, a 53-year-old male, underwent renal transplantation approximately 10 hours ago. Stat Doppler examination was requested and demonstrated an absence of venous flow and marked vascular impedance within the transplant. The possible cause is:
A. pyelonephritis.
B. renal vein thrombosis.
C. acute tubular necrosis.
D. lymphocele development.

65. Color Doppler relies heavily on filters because:
A. it samples multiple points at a very fast rate.
B. all but continuously moving signals must be eliminated.
C. it operates at only 60 frames/s.
D. it is subject to grating lobes.

66. Occlusion of the internal carotid artery over a long period of time may cause:
A. extreme turbulence.
B. enlargement of the external carotid.
C. difficulties in vessel identification.
D. B and C

67. Which of the following statements concerning continuous wave Doppler is *untrue?*
    A. Lacks axial resolution
    B. May use filters to decrease noise interference
    C. May use a quadrature phase detector
    D. Is useful in determining vessel depth

68. Heterogeneous plaque accompanied by cystic or hypoechoic areas within the carotid artery usually indicate the presence of:
    A. intraplaque hemorrhage.
    B. ulcerations secondary to plaque.
    C. an acute inflammatory response.
    D. a postsurgical complication.

69. Testicular artery flow characteristically demonstrates:
    A. low peripheral resistance.
    B. high peripheral resistance.
    C. narrow systolic peaks.
    D. low diastolic flow.

70. Select the *false* statement about aliasing.
    A. Does not occur with continuous-wave Doppler
    B. Occurs at the Nyquist limit in pulsed-wave and color Doppler
    C. May appear as concurrent reversed flow
    D. All of the above

71. Doppler flow patterns vary because of patient respiratory changes. Flow _____ during inspiration and _____ with expiration.
    A. decreases; increases
    B. increases; decreases
    C. increases; remains constant
    D. remains constant; decreases

72. A patient with massive deep vein thrombosis of the legs above the femoral artery level is best managed by _____ to prevent pulmonary thromboembolism.
    A. aspirin therapy
    B. heparin therapy
    C. insertion of a Greenfield filter
    D. B and C

73. The risk factors for DVT following major general surgery are:
    A. patients who do not take aspirin.
    B. age, malignancy, obesity, and the presence of varicose veins.
    C. lengthy surgery, history of DVT, and diabetes.
    D. B and C

74. Venous plethysmography methods that are helpful include:
    A. strain gauges.
    B. pneumatic plethysmography.
    C. impedance transducers.
    D. all of the above

75. Venous plethysmography techniques are used to measure:
    A. arterial and venous pressure.
    B. venous capacitance.
    C. venous outflow volume changes.
    D. B and C

76. A venous plotted index nomo-
    graph reads:
    A. frequency.
    B. ohms.
    C. velocity.
    D. megaHertz.

77. Reduced accuracy of spectral
    analysis Doppler signals from
    the carotid arteries was a prob-
    lem in the past, until recog-
    nition of the hemodynamic
    principles of _____ were
    studied.
    A. blood pressure
    B. cardiac output
    C. contralateral high grade or
       occluded carotid arteries
    D. none of the above

78. The external iliac arteries sup-
    ply the leg and become the
    common femoral arteries at ap-
    proximately the level of the:
    A. profunda femoris.
    B. iliac crest.
    C. inguinal ligament.
    D. buttocks.

79. Which of the following symp-
    toms are seen in patients with
    advancing peripheral vascular
    arterial disease?

A. Erythema
B. Dependent rubor or eleva-
   tion pallor
C. Thickened nails
D. All of the above

80. Normal arterial flow signals are
    said to be _____; with arterial
    obstruction the flow signal be-
    comes _____.
    A. biphasic; triphasic
    B. triphasic; biphasic or
       monophasic
    C. monophasic; biphasic or
       triphasic
    D. biphasic; monophasic

81. Thoracic outlet syndrome usu-
    ally involves the:
    A. subclavian artery.
    B. subclavian vein.
    C. brachial nerve plexus.
    D. all of the above

82. Patients who present with vas-
    cular spasms or obstruction
    related to cold and abrupt tem-
    perature changes are most
    likely to suffer from:
    A. Buerger's disease.
    B. Marfan's syndrome.
    C. Reynaud's phenomenon.
    D. frostbite.

CASES AND QUESTIONS

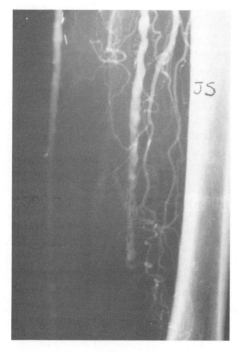

Figure 7-1. Venogram. (Courtesy of William G. Hayden, M.D., Sequoia Hospital, Redwood City, California.)

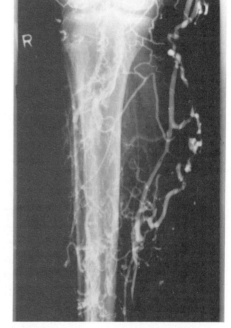

Figure 7-2. Venogram. (Courtesy of William G. Hayden, M.D., Sequoia Hospital, Redwood City, California.)

83. Figure 7-1 is an arteriogram of the lower extremity demonstrating:
    A. obstruction of the greater saphenous (GSV) vein.
    B. a normal saphenofemoral graft with occlusion of the SFA.
    C. a normal superficial femoral artery (SFA).
    D. a normal arteriogram of the lower extremity.

84. The venogram presented in Figure 7-2 demonstrates:
    A. normal popliteal veins.
    B. normal veins of the lower extremity.
    C. extensive deep vein thrombosis (DVT) of the popliteal vein and calf veins.
    D. an abnormal greater saphenous vein in the groin.

85. Plate 7-1 demonstrates a _____ , originating at the bifurcation of the femoral artery.
    A. hematoma
    B. venous varicosity
    C. Dale shunt
    D. false aneurysm

86. Plate 7-2 represents an example of a Dale shunt within the femoral vein. The purpose of using a Dale shunt is to:
    A. prevent varicosities by decreasing flow to the veins.
    B. reduce the chance of venous thrombus by increasing the velocity of venous flow.
    C. reduce arterial pressure by shunting blood from the femoral artery.
    D. increase venous pressure.

87. Identify the abnormality demonstrated in Plate 7-3.
    A. Severe kinking of internal carotid artery
    B. Loop with retroverted flow
    C. Minor kinking of the left internal carotid artery
    D. Normal finding post endarterectomy

88. Plate 7-4 presents an example of a:
    A. superficial femoral artery stenosis.
    B. superficial femoral artery, small branch.
    C. complete obstruction of the superficial femoral artery.
    D. normal superficial femoral artery.

89. The Doppler spectral analysis of the femoral artery presented in Plate 7-5 is:
    A. normal.
    B. triphasic.
    C. monophasic.
    D. multiphasic.

90. The carotid artery plaque seen in Plate 7-6 should be classified as:
    A. homogeneous.
    B. a 10% stenosis.
    C. heterogeneous.
    D. a 50% stenosis.

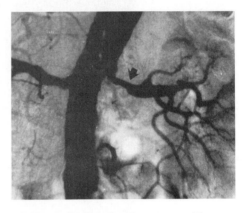

Figure 7-3. Renal arteriogram. (Courtesy of William G. Hayden, M.D., Sequoia Hospital, Redwood City, California.)

91. Figure 7-3 represents a substraction arteriogram of a:
    A. normal renal transplant artery.
    B. stenosis of the left renal artery.
    C. short segment stenosis of the right renal artery.
    D. site of anastamosis of the left renal artery in a transplanted kidney.

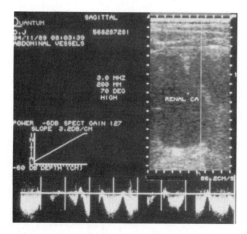

Figure 7-4. Renal tumor scan. (Courtesy of David B. Smith, M.D., Good Samaritan Hospital, San Jose, California.)

92. The renal tumor depicted in Figure 7-4 in addition demonstrates a:
    A. normal left renal artery.
    B. normal phasicity of the inferior vena cava (IVC).
    C. distal portion of a normal renal vein.
    D. distal portion of an abnormal renal vein caused by tumor complication.

93. Patients are always referred for investigation of the _____ prior to removal of renal tumors.
    A. inferior vena cava (IVC)
    B. IVC and renal veins
    C. IVC and portal veins
    D. aorta, renal arteries, and IVC

94. Access veins (see Plate 7-7) demonstrate:
    A. normal flow.
    B. high-velocity arterial and venous flow.
    C. high-velocity arterial flow.
    D. abnormally high venous flow velocities.

95. The purpose of an access vein is to:
    A. shunt blood to the hand.
    B. provide a puncture site for renal dialysis.
    C. provide routine intravenous punctures.
    D. provide better blood pressure readings.

96. Obstruction of an arm access vein:
    A. is dangerous because renal dialysis function occurs at this site and does not circulate to the rest of the body.
    B. will produce difficulties in dialysis needle insertion.
    C. seldom occurs.
    D. presents no danger, since the use of an access vein is permissable even when it is occluded.

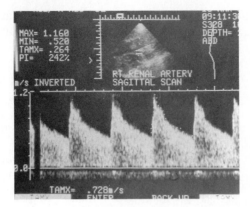

Figure 7-5. Renal artery scan.

97. Figure 7-5 represents a right renal artery stenosis. The renal artery is depicted:
   A. in cross-section, posterior to the inferior vena cava, as seen on a sagittal scan with the patient lying in the lateral decubitus position.
   B. as a sagittal oblique scan with the length of the vessel and is located posterior to the inferior vena cava.
   C. cannot be seen at all in a sagittal scan.
   D. represents the right renal artery, lying anterior to the inferior vena cava.

98. Select the correct equation or procedure for the diagnosis of renal artery stenosis.
   A. Renal artery systolic velocity/diastolic velocity
   B. The pulsatility index
   C. Highest renal artery velocity/aortic velocity taken at the level of the superior mesenteric artery
   D. Highest renal stenotic velocity/the velocity of renal artery flow taken in the

normal kidney (at the origin of its renal artery)

99. The diastolic component of the renal artery waveform seen in Figure 7-5 increases with renal disease because:
   A. the artery is less compliant.
   B. renal failure has occurred.
   C. of combined aortic disease.
   D. the opposing renal artery is obstructed.

100. Plate 7-8 is a cross-sectional scan demonstrating the right common carotid artery with the jugular vein lying anterior and lateral. The jugular vein in this scan is:
   A. not well-visualized because of failure to perform a Valsalva maneuver.
   B. thrombosed.
   C. normal.
   D. ectatic.

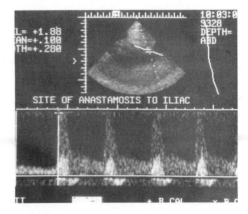

Figure 7-6. Renal transplant.

101. The duplex scan in Figure 7-6 was taken following kidney transplantation. The spectrum demonstrates:

A. the external iliac artery.

B. the renal artery anastomotic site aliasing.

C. the renal artery anastomotic site and the external iliac artery.

D. the highest velocity is the renal artery anastomosis site; the lowest velocity is the internal iliac artery.

102. The sample gate cursor seen in Plate 7-9 is placed within the left renal artery. Identify the vessel lying directly above it.

A. Splenic vein

B. Left renal vein

C. Dilated gastric vein (varicosity)

D. Dilated pancreatic duct

103. Accurate spectral analysis of the interlobar and arcuate arteries (see Plate 7-10) requires adjustment of the baseline velocity scale to:

A. medium flow, allowing higher velocities since the vessels are smaller in diameter.

B. higher flow, since smaller vessels possess higher velocities.

C. medium or slower sampling because of renal insufficiency.

D. higher flow for better color-flow saturation.

104. The diagnosis of renal transplant rejection or renal failure can be made upon:

A. studying the renal origins and all renal branches and calculating their pulsatility index or resistant index.

B. dividing the highest renal artery velocities by the aortic velocity.

C. observing the main renal artery and the interlobular arteries within the renal pelvis.

D. none of the above

105. Identify the abdominal vessel indicated by the arrows in Plate 7-11.

A. Stenotic iliac artery

B. Inferior mesenteric artery

C. Inferior gastric artery

D. "Wandering artery of Drummond"

106. Plate 7-12 represents a cross-sectional view of:

A. an old venous thrombus.

B. a recent deep thrombotic event.

C. postthrombotic syndrome in the leg.

D. partial occlusion of the popliteal vein.

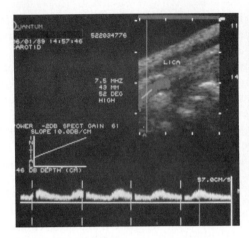

Figure 7-7. Sagittal cross-sectional color-flow scan.

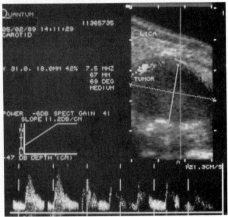

Figure 7-8. Carotid artery tumor.

107. Plate 7-13 demonstrates the internal carotid artery in red, and the external carotid artery in blue. A patent vertebral artery was also demonstrated in cross-section and sagittal scan (Fig. 7-7). In order for this to occur:
    A. the external carotid artery will display diastole shorter than that of the internal carotid artery.
    B. the external carotid artery is retrograde.
    C. the common carotid artery must be chronically occluded, with the external carotid artery supplying the internal carotid artery.
    D. B and C.

108. A rare, carotid body tumor is located posterior to the internal carotid artery in Figure 7-8. Which of the following statements concerning this mass is *true*?
    A. The internal flow is normal
    B. The internal flow of this carotid body tumor is mildly resistant
    C. The carotid tumor is occluding the internal carotid artery, distally
    D. None of the above

109. The terminal aorta flow pattern seen in Plate 7-14:
    A. more resistant than the upper abdominal portion of the aorta because the lower extremity arteries are more resistant.
    B. nonresistant throughout.
    C. triphasic at the terminal portion in young patients.
    D. A and C

110. The internal carotid artery displayed in Plate 7-15 is:
    A. mildly kinked, accompanied by mild distal turbulence.
    B. moderately kinked, accompanied by increased velocity and mild turbulence distally.
    C. moderately kinked, and increased velocity should be demonstrated by velocity spectral analysis.
    D. normal.

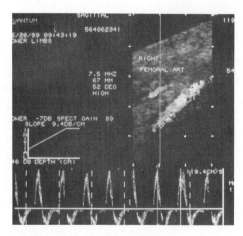

Figure 7-9. Right femoral artery scan.

111. Doppler study of the common femoral artery seen in Figure 7-9 should be:
    A. sampled at the inguinal ligament.
    B. biphasic with a 35–55° angle.
    C. retrograde at the profunda junction.
    D. sampled 2–3 cm above the bifurcation of the superficial femoral artery and profunda.

112. The waveform demonstrated in Plate 7-16 is greater than 70% stenotic. The "B." 75.59 represents:
    A. diastolic velocity.
    B. peak systolic velocity that is aliasing.
    C. a problem with the PRF.
    D. B and C

113. Plate 7-17 demonstrates a:
    A. superficial femoral vein valve.
    B. residual flow coming down the leg.
    C. residual lumen proximal to the superficial femoral vein.
    D. none of the above

114. In Plate 7-18, thickening of the walls of either deep or superficial veins is a sign of:
    A. advancing age.
    B. an old DVT (deep venous thrombosis).
    C. a new thrombus.
    D. normalcy.

115. In Plate 7-19 partial occlusion of the superficial femoral vein:
    A. requires no treatment because the superficial femoral is not a deep vein and will not cause a pulmonary embolus.
    B. will never become fully occluded as the result of venous pressure.
    C. and occluded veins both require the same treatment.
    D. all of the above

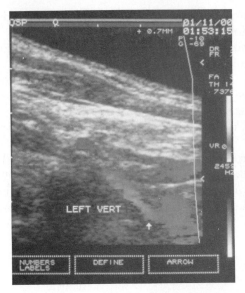

Figure 7-10. Scan of the left vertebral artery.

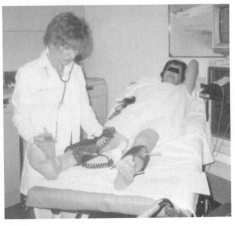

Figure 7-11. Vascular examination procedure.

116. Figure 7-10 demonstrates the left vertebral artery origin. The vessel seen to the far right on this scan is the:
    A. aortic arch.
    B. innominate artery.
    C. subclavian vein.
    D. subclavian artery.

117. Figure 7-11 demonstrates the proper procedure during:
    A. a venous exam using audible Doppler.
    B. waveform and artery pressure of the dorsalis pedis artery.
    C. postexercise pressure readings to diagnose claudication.
    D. air plethysmography for arterial disease.

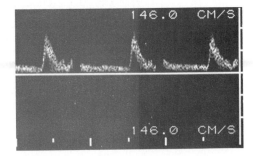

Figure 7-12. Spectral analysis scan.

118. Figure 7-12 demonstrates the spectrum of the:

A. splenic vein reversed.
B. external carotid artery.
C. common carotid artery.
D. femoral artery.

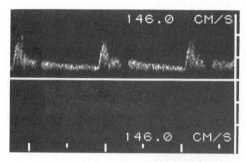

Figure 7-13. Arterial spectral analysis.

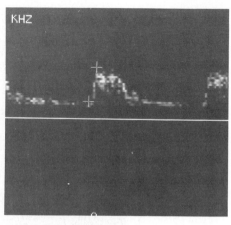

Figure 7-15. Arterial scan.

119. Identify the extracranial vessel seen in Figure 7-13.
    A. Internal carotid artery
    B. External carotid artery
    C. Vertebral artery
    D. Temporal artery

121. Identify the extracranial arterial vessel seen in Figure 7-15.
    A. External carotid artery
    B. "Dampened" external carotid artery
    C. Common carotid artery damped because of proximal or distal disease
    D. Normal abdominal aorta

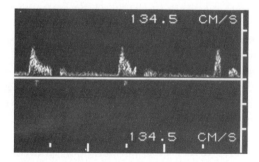

Figure 7-14. Arterial spectral analysis.

120. Figure 7-14 demonstrates the:
    A. internal carotid artery.
    B. external carotid artery.
    C. femoral artery.
    D. common carotid artery.

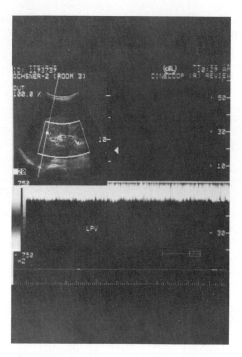

Figure 7-16. Longitudinal scan of the liver with Doppler sampling of the left portal vein. (Courtesy of Benita Barthel, R.T., R.D.M.S., Ochsner Medical Foundation, New Orleans, Louisiana.)

This patient is a 58-year-old white male with a long history of alcohol abuse (30-plus years, at 1 quart a day), diagnosed with hepatic cirrhosis. He presents with fatigue, anorexia, edema, ascites, and hepatic encephalopathy and malnutrition. The BUN, creatinine, PT, and PTT liver function tests were elevated. The patient has a past history of aortorenal shunt due to a left renal artery stenosis, and was being considered for a liver transplant. Abdominal ultrasound studies revealed findings consistent with moderate ascites, forward flow in the hepatic veins, IVC, and hepatic artery. Reversed flow was observed in the portal vein with an increase in collateral flow from the hepatic artery. The liver was very attenuative. The spleen, while not significantly enlarged, contained multiple collaterals. The gallbladder was normal and, although no hydronephrosis was seen, the right kidney contained an incidental lower-pole cyst of approximately 2 cm in diameter. The patient was subsequently determined not to be a liver transplant candidate at this time.

122. The Doppler evaluation of the left portal vein in Figure 7-16 demonstrates:
    A. normal flow.
    B. reversed flow.
    C. triphasic flow.
    D. no flow.

123. If blood flow is described as *hepatopedal*, then it:
    A. flows toward the liver.
    B. flows away from the liver.
    C. is considered reversed flow.
    D. is considered collateral flow.

124. Reversal of the portal vein blood flow may result from all except:
    A. Budd-Chiari syndrome.
    B. occlusion of a portacaval shunt.
    C. cirrhosis of the liver.
    D. right ventricular failure.

125. Low portal vein flow velocity has been found to be a useful indicator of:
    A. deteriorating liver function.

B. normal liver function.

C. occlusion of the portal vein.

D. detection of hepatic tumors.

126. The portal vein flow pattern with normal respiration is:

A. biphasic.

B. triphasic.

C. continuous.

D. none of the above

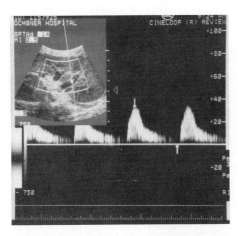

Figure 7-17. Renal transplant. (Courtesy of Jeanie Marchese, Ochsner Medical Foundation, New Orleans, Louisiana.)

The patient was a 44-year-old white male diabetic with a recent third renal transplant and simultaneous first pancreatic transplant. The patient complains of diarrhea, abdominal distention, and decreased urine output. Laboratory studies revealed elevated levels of BUN, creatinine, uric acid, and glucose. Ultrasound findings were free-fluid around the pancreatic transplant. The kidney transplant spectrum demonstrated

significant loss of diastolic flow, suggesting the possibility of cyclosporine toxicity versus rejection. No other studies were performed to confirm renal transplant rejection.

127. The image in Figure 7-17 represents a Doppler waveform signal obtained from the renal artery of a transplant patient. The resistive index value is 1.00. What is the formula used to obtain this value?

A. $\dfrac{\text{systolic peak} + \text{end diastolic peak}}{\text{systolic peak}}$

B. $\dfrac{\text{systolic peak}}{\text{diastolic peak}}$

C. $\dfrac{\text{systolic peak} - \text{diastolic peak}}{\text{systolic peak}}$

D. $\dfrac{\text{diastolic peak} - \text{systolic peak}}{\text{systolic peak}}$

128. A resistive index of _____ is considered normal.

A. .80

B. .45

C. .95

D. 1.00

129. Doppler sampling of the _____ artery is considered the most sensitive location to determine renal transplant rejection using a resistive index.

A. main renal

B. anastomic site

C. segmental

D. interlobular

130. The most common complication indicated by an abnormal resistive index value may

indicate all of the following *except:*
A. renal artery stenosis.
B. hydronephrosis.
C. rejection.
D. cyclosporine toxicity.

131. Renal transplants are surgically placed within the:
A. femoral fossa.
B. native kidney fossa.
C. iliac fossa.
D. inferior mesenteric artery origin.

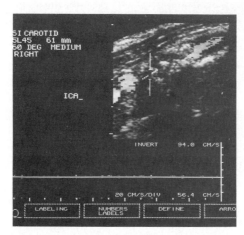

Figure 7-18. Longitudinal image of right internal carotid artery and corresponding Doppler spectral analysis. (Courtesy of Dixie Alexander, Ochsner Medical Foundation, New Orleans, Louisiana.)

This patient is an 82-year-old white male with a history of coronary artery bypass graft surgery, bilateral prostatic hypertrophy (BPH), blindness in the right eye due to glaucoma, peripheral vascular disease, bilateral carotid occlusion, and COPD. He has bilateral carotid bruits R > L. The patient is currently doing well, with no surgeries performed. Carotid artery studies found complete occlusion of the right internal carotid artery, with some flow in the right common and external carotid arteries and the presence of plaque. Complete occlusion of the left internal, external carotid artery and bulb, with blunted flow in the left common carotid artery, was noted. Forward flow was present in both vertebral arteries. Flow was also seen in both subclavian arteries without obvious stenosis. No other studies were performed to confirm the ultrasound diagnosis.

132. Doppler sampling of the internal carotid artery in Figure 7-18 concludes a diagnosis of:
A. normal internal carotid artery.
B. ectatic internal carotid artery.
C. probable occluded internal carotid artery.
D. turbulence in the internal carotid artery.

133. With internal carotid artery occlusion, _____ may be mistaken for the internal carotid artery.
A. branches of the external carotid artery
B. branches of the common carotid artery
C. the vertebral artery
D. branches of the subclavian artery

134. Where is(are) the most common site(s) for plaque forma-

tion in the extracranial carotid system?
A. Distal portion of the internal carotid artery
B. Origin of the internal carotid artery
C. The carotid bifurcation
D. B and C

135. How is flow affected in the common carotid artery when an internal carotid artery occlusion is present?
A. Normal diastolic flow
B. Increased diastolic flow
C. Decreased diastolic flow
D. Increased systolic and diastolic flow

136. To help distinguish between the internal carotid artery and the external carotid artery in cases of internal artery occlusion with Doppler, sonographers should:
A. finger-tap the area over the vertebral artery.
B. finger-tap the area over the temporal artery.
C. finger-tap the area of the common carotid artery.
D. do nothing.

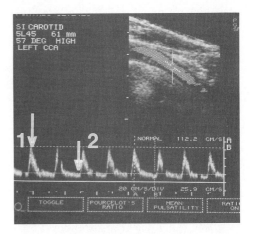

Figure 7-19. Longitudinal left common carotid artery scan. (Courtesy of Jeanie Marchese, Ochsner Medical Foundation, New Orleans, Louisiana.)

This 82-year-old male patient had symptomatic angina with vigorous exercise. He had a positive treadmill test at Stage 1. Cardiac catheterization found significant three-vessel coronary artery disease. Ultrasound studies of the carotid arteries demonstrated 80% to 90% stenosis of the right internal carotid artery and 80% to 90% stenosis of the left internal carotid artery. The patient underwent coronary artery bypass surgery and a left endarterectomy.

137. The Doppler spectral analysis of the left common carotid artery in Figure 7-19 indicates:
A. normal flow.
B. reversed flow.
C. total occlusion.
D. turbulent flow.

138. Arrow 1 indicates the _____ portion of the Doppler waveform.
A. baseline
B. systolic

C. diastolic

D. reversed

139. Arrow 2 indicates the _____ portion of the Doppler waveform.

A. baseline

B. systolic

C. diastolic

D. reversed

140. A typical Doppler waveform of the external carotid artery demonstrates a lower velocity in diastole, indicating:

A. high-resistance circulation.

B. low-impedance circulation.

C. vascular stasis.

D. occlusion of the distal external carotid artery.

ANSWERS

1. A. The audible range of Doppler shift frequencies falls between 200 Hertz to 15 kiloHertz.[9]

2. D. The color priority or gray scale control determines whether gray scale or color Doppler information will be emphasized. This same control also can be used to increase or decrease color saturation, and as a filter, by suppressing color information above a certain operator-set level.[9]

3. D. The adductor (Hunter's) canal lies in the middle and lower third of the thigh, immediately distal to the apex of the femoral triangle. It is an intermuscular cleft situated beneath the sartorius muscle and is bounded laterally by the vastus medialis muscle and posteriorly by the adductor longus and magnus muscles. It contains the femoral vessels and the saphenous nerve.[25]

4. C. A 0 degree angle causes the greatest Doppler shift. Degree of angle is a function of cosine theda in the Doppler shift equation.

5. B. At approximately the level of the thyroid cartilage, the common carotid artery bifurcates into a more anteromedial external carotid artery and a more posterolateral internal carotid artery.[9, 25]

6. D. One of the color Doppler controls governs the number of cycles per color line and is referred to as dwell time, ensemble length, or packet size. If this control is increased, flow sensitivity increases, but frame rate decreases.[16]

7. A. PW Doppler suffers from such poor signal-to-noise ratios that it may be difficult to detect low flow signals because of noise interference.[8, 15, 29]

8. D. Associated risk factors for atherosclerotic disease are cigarette smoking, diabetes, hypertension, hyperlipidemia or hypercholesterolosis, a family history of diabetes with peripheral neuropathy, falsely elevated ABIs, and atherosclerotic disease.[16, 26]

9. B. The superficial femoral vein follows a medial course along the inner curve of the thigh "in seam," and at its inferior aspect, just superior to the knee, lies posterior to the superficial femoral artery.[8, 9]

10. B. Green is the color most often chosen to display the highest velocity ranges.[9]

11. C. In a study by Fleischer et al., ovarian malignancies demonstrated relatively slow flow and lack of a diastolic notch. The latter is probably related to the lack or scarcity of smooth muscle in the tumor vessels. Malignant lesions tended to have central areas of abnormal vessels.[4,7]

12. D. Valves are commonly seen in the larger veins to prevent the back flow of blood. These are often seen in the greater saphenous vein and its collaterals, the common femoral vein and the superficial femoral vein, and sometimes within the popliteal veins.[8,9,25]

13. B. Patient complaints of a sensation of cramping or burning pain, or "tiredness" of the calf, thigh, and buttocks related to exercise are the most frequently described symptoms of intermittent claudication involving the iliac arteries to the calf. The site or level of the cramping is related to the arteries that are diseased.[6]

14. B. Abdominal masses or low-flow vessels often demonstrate a spectral appearance of lower systolic peaks and a more pronounced diastolic component.[9]

15. C. The carotid arteries are located medial to the internal jugular vein, lateral to the thyroid gland, and posteromedial to the sternocleidomastoid muscle.[8,9]

16. A. Continuous-wave systems are more consistently sensitive in detecting areas of flow, including smaller tumor vessels with multidirectional flow.[4,8]

17. A. Hepatic arteries are associated with a low-impedance flow and a high-diastolic complement.[9]

18. D. The missed diagnosis of occlusion can result from mistaking the internal for the external or external branch for the internal carotid artery. Shadowing caused by plaque mineralization, poor vessel tortuosity, poor scanning techniques, or weak returning Doppler signals distal to a point of extreme stenosis are other contributing factors.[16]

19. C. With spectral analysis, the Doppler signal is displayed in such a way that the power or intensity of each velocity is assigned a shade of gray.[9]

20. C. A drop in pressure of 20 to 30 mm/hg between segments indicates an element of occlusive disease in the intervening segment. A drop of 10 (ankle/arm index B) is diagnostic for occlusive disease.[16]

21. D. Proper evaluation of the lower-extremity arteries requires 3 to 4 cuffs. The fourth cuff is used for an ankle pressure if the patient is diabetic.[21]

22. A. Adequate evaluation in the Hunter's canal region can be difficult due to the depth of the vessels relative to transducer function. A lower transducer megahertz is helpful for this area.[16]

23. B. Fresh thrombus is hypoechoic with vessel wall enlargement, while chronic thrombus of several months or years results in reduced vessel diameter and an echogenic pattern. Internal echoes begin to occur in fresh thrombus within 6 to 8 hours.[21]

24. D. The colors used for Doppler display are based on three characteristics: hue (primarily colors of red, blue, and green are used), saturation (amount of white present in a color), and luminosity (the brightness of a color).[16]

25. D. Photoplethysmography can be useful in evaluating small-vessel disease such as diabetes and vasospastic disorders. The technique employs application of a small, light-sensitive transducer directly to the toes to detect cutaneous blood flow. The recordings are similar to those described for volume plethysmographic tracings and documents relative perfusion of the digits studied.[16]

26. C. In venous hypertension, the splanchnic veins will dilate to diameters greater than 1.5 cm.[9, 23, 25]

27. C

28. B

29. E

30. D

31. A[8, 9]

32. B. Peripheral vascular scanning is ideally performed with either a 5- or 7-MHz linear-array transducer, with Doppler or color Doppler capabilities.[9, 16]

33. C. The Doppler shift decreases as the Doppler angle increases. Usually operator-controlled, the angle should be set between 45 and 60 degrees to ensure the best conversion in the velocity equation.[8, 9]

34. C. Fetal Doppler examination of the fetal heart and umbilical cord has been approved by the American Institute of Ultrasound in Medicine (AIUM), whenever it is clinically indicated.[9, 16]

35. A. A resting patient should have an ankle/arm index (AAI) of 1.0. A common technical error involves falsely lowering ankle pressures in patients with a slower than normal heart rate. This usually occurs when the pressure gauge is released too rapidly, missing the correct return systolic pressure.[22]

36. C. Normally, the blood flow in the portal vein is steady. The presence of respiratory variations (biphasic signals) suggests portal hypertension. This is due to increased resistance. It is important, however, to differentiate portal vein branches from dilated biliary ducts.[8, 27]

37. C. Typically, normal Doppler arterial signals in a lower extremity are triphasic. The key components are a brisk upstroke and rapid downstroke, with a slight negative component, followed by an additional positive component of the signal corresponding to some forward arterial flow during diastole.[8, 16, 27]

38. C. Sampling should be complete throughout the entire vessel, but peak velocities are most likely to be encountered midvessel, and any velocity samples taken for calculations should be taken at midvessel. Color flow is the best guide in a narrow vessel.[27]

39. D. Each vein should be examined for the presence or absence of an intraluminal mass, the compressibility of the vein, the resting, augmented Doppler signal intensities, and color-flow mapping of vessel lumens.[8, 27]

40. D. Aliasing may occur in color Doppler systems as an abrupt color change (not caused by flow reversal) within the same vessel. It is often seen as a change in high-frequency color codes (e.g., light red to light blue).[27]

41. A. Normal renal artery resistance is a peak velocity of <100 cm/s (persistently decreasing diastolic flow due to low resistance).[12, 13, 19]

42. B. Vascular rejection, which is usually not seen until the second week after surgery, results in an endovasculitis with small vessel thrombosis and diffuse white blood cell infiltration.[19]

43. D. Immediately after exercise, ankle and brachial pressures and ankle plethysmography are repeated and compared to preexercise studies. The expected response postexercise is an elevation of brachial and ankle pressures above resting levels, with ABIs remaining stable.[16]

44. D. A Valsalva maneuver is used to assess valve competence.[8,9,27]

45. C. Abnormal plethysmographic recordings may become degraded in morphology and amplitude. The indications are characteristic broadening and decreased amplitude of the tracings and the loss of the dicrotic notch. Just as the tracings indicate perfusion of the segment measured, degradation implies disease of the inflow to that segment.[6]

46. B. The infraorbital artery is a terminal branch of the maxillary artery.

47. C. The current clinical role of Doppler ultrasound is to detect vascular patterns consistent with tumor activity. Doppler signals are reasonably specific for malignancy, but not particularly sensitive. Even if sensitivity improved, Doppler imaging of breast vascularity would be limited because study of the whole breast takes so long to perform.[4]

48. B. If the Doppler angle is set at 90°, or perpendicular to flow, the computer will be unable to detect forward from reverse flow.[8,9,27]

49. B. Grating lobes result from decreased lateral resolution because the beam is not perpendicular to the target. To correct, the transducer angle or Doppler steering angle should be adjusted.[8,9,27]

50. C. Veins possess thin walls comprised of three layers: the outermost layer (tunica adventitia), the middle layer (tunica media), and the inner layer (intima).[8,9,23–25]

51. D. Yellow, white, or mosaic patterns represent high-velocity or complex-flow patterns.[3,9,10]

52. B. To correct mirror image or range ambiguity artifacts, the PRF and far gain should be decreased and the frequency of the transducer should be increased.[8,9]

53. B

54. C

55. A

56. E

57. D^{16}

58. B. Color Doppler systems are unable to detect flow less than approximately 0.06 m/s.[27]

59. D. Cellulitis, the general inflammation of the skin and interstitial tissues of the leg, may make deep vein visualization difficult because of the inflammation present, and the increased echogenicity it produces. An IPG or a venogram is an alternative.[16,27]

60. B. Varicoceles are often easily visualized. During Valsalva maneuvers the observation of a vein greater than 3 mm in diameter is considered evidence of a varicocele.[27]

61. B. Stenotic plaque should be measured in the transverse plane to ensure highest accuracy. Additional images of plaque may be necessary; it is important to look for irregularities along the borders of plaque, which may indicate the presence of ulcerations.[8,9,27]

62. D. With renal transplant rejection there is often decreased blood flow due to decreased renal function (often due to external compression or narrowing of smaller blood vessels). There will also be decreased diastolic flow.[9,12,19,27]

63. C. During the follicular phases of ovulation, diastolic flow normally decreases.[7,23,27]

64. B. In the immediate postoperative period, abnormal vascular impedance is usually due to renal vein thrombosis. After 24 hours, causes include acute tubular necrosis, obstruction, pyelonephritis, and extrarenal compression.[19]

65. A. Color Doppler offers a display of mean flow velocities (spatially) by sampling multiple points at a very fast rate. Multiple sampling often causes noise from tissue movement as well as from moving blood signals. Filters must be used to eliminate all but the continuously moving signals.[14,16,27]

66. D. Long-standing occlusion of the internal carotid artery may cause

enlargement of the external carotid artery and its branches, which may in turn cause erroneous vessel identification.[15, 16, 27]

67. D. Continuous-wave Doppler techniques cannot determine vessel depth.[8, 9, 27]

68. A. Heterogeneous plaque with cystic or hyperechoic areas is considered an indication of the presence of intraplaque hemorrhage.[15, 18]

69. A. The testicular artery has low peripheral resistance with broad systolic peaks and high diastolic flow.[23, 27]

70. D. Aliasing does not occur with continuous-wave Doppler, but does occur in pulsed-wave and color Doppler at the Nyquist limit. The maximum frequency level that can be displayed is equal to $\frac{1}{2}$ of the system's PRF. If the Doppler frequency exceeds that level, aliasing will occur. An aliased signal will wrap around the baseline or may appear as concurrent reversed flow.[27]

71. A. Phasicity is the term used to describe Doppler flow pattern variations due to patient respiratory changes. There will be decreases in flow with inspiration, followed by increased flow with expiration.[3, 9, 23, 27]

72. D. The Greenfield filter is a stainless-steel device inserted into the inferior vena cava through the jugular or common femoral vein. It has been clinically proven effective in the mechanical prevention of pulmonary thromboembolism. Some patients may require heparin to prevent small emboli passing through the filter.[14]

73. D. The risk factors for DVT are often great when the patient has several predisposing conditions such as a malignancy, history of DVT, obesity, diabetes, varicose veins, and with advancing age.[17]

74. D[17]

75. D. Venous plethysmography is used to measure venous capacitance and outflow volume change.[17]

76. B. Venous function index nomographs employ the use of ohms.[17]

77. C. It has been postulated that the improved accuracy of Doppler spectral analysis is due to an understanding of the hemodynamic effects of the ipsilateral stenosis, with compensatory increased flow resulting in elevated peak systolic frequencies in the contralateral vessel.[18]

78. C. The iliac artery becomes the common femoral artery at approximately the level of the inguinal ligament.[2]

79. D. Erythema is often seen in patients with advancing arterial disease, along with drying and flaking of the skin and thickening of the nails. If an extremity is held dependently it will usually present puffy and reddened; upon limb elevation, the redness will disappear and the limb will become very pale.[2]

80. B. The normal arterial flow signal is comprised of three components, and is said to be triphasic. In cases of arterial obstruction the flow signal begins to lose one or more components, becoming biphasic or monophasic.[2]

81. D. Thoracic outlet syndrome occurs when the arteries, veins, or nerves supplying the arm are obstructed by compression between the clavicle and first rib, a cervical rib and the scalene muscles, or the pectoralis minor with hyperabduction of the arm. The vessels usually involved are the subclavian artery and vein and the brachial nerve plexus where it leaves the chest and goes to the arm.[2]

82. C. Reynaud's phenomenon is related to cold and abrupt temperature changes, which cause vascular spasm in the digits and resulting obstruction. Purplish fingers and toes are often seen with this disorder. It is often seen in patients with lupus erythematosis, arthritis, and other diseases.[2]

83. B. The saphenous vein was used to bypass the occluded SFA by stripping the valves of the saphenous vein or placing it *in situ*.

84. C. An extra, irregular collateral varicosity appears off the right greater saphenous vein. There is extensive deep vein thrombosis of the lower leg.[3]

85. D. This patient suffered a false aneurysm, which developed following arterial puncture (via the femoral artery) for cardiac arteriography and percutaneous transluminal angioplasty (PTA).[11]

86. B. Dale shunts are commonly used in an attempt to reduce the formation of venous thrombus by increasing the velocity of venous flow.[21]

87. A. Plate 7-3 represents severe kinking of the internal carotid artery (ICA). This type of kinking causes turbulent arterial flow.[21]

88. A. Superficial femoral artery stenosis is demonstrated by the narrowing of the vessel and the vascular turbulence demonstrated by color Doppler. The superficial femoral vein (SFV) is seen posterior to the artery.[21]

89. C. A single curve displayed on the spectral analysis with a pulsatility index of 1.0 to 1.2 indicates severe iliac artery disease.[2]

90. C. A plaque that is composed of calcium and fat is heterogeneous.[10]

91. B. In general, any lesion longer than 1/2 cm is considered long segmented.[2,12]

92. C. It is important to demonstrate a tumor-free IVC and renal veins.

93. B. Duplex color-flow is often performed prior to nephrectomy to rule out tumor invasion of the renal veins and the inferior vena cava.[9,29]

94. B[1,12,21]

95. B[21]

96. A. The dialysis process takes place within the arm access vein and does not circulate to the rest of the body.[21]

97. A. The scan demonstrates a cross-sectional view of the renal artery as it lies posterior to the inferior vena cava. This type of image is achieved when the patient lies in the lateral decubitus position.[12]

98. C. The equation for the diagnosis of renal artery stenosis is the highest renal artery velocity divided by the aortic velocity at the level of the superior mesenteric artery.[12]

99. A. The diastolic velocity increases in the renal artery and internal carotid stenoses.

100. B. The jugular vein shows evidence of thrombus. Investigation of the subclavian vein for thrombosis was also indicated in this patient, who had multiple needle sticks to the jugular vein.[2]

101. D. The sample gate can be closed after detection of renal artery flow to eliminate the iliac artery signal.[2,12]

102. B. At the origin of the renal arteries, the left and right renal veins lie anterior to the artery.[28]

103. C. The higher the patient's BUN and creatinine levels, the less blood will flow to the kidneys, regardless of vessel diameters.[21]

104. A. It is important to study the entire upper-, mid-, and lower-pole interlobular and arcuate vessels, since infarct will occlude flow to one portion of the kidney.[13]

105. B[28]

106. B. The increased size of the vein is indicative of a recent deep venous thrombotic (DVT) event.[21]

107. D. The external branches of the carotid are supplying the external carotid artery, making it retrograde, and the internal carotid artery is prograde. The distal common carotid artery is occluded.[21]

108. B. Carotid body tumors are extremely rare and a vascular surgeon may see only one case in his or her entire career. The flow is mildly resistant, indicating that the diastolic velocity should be higher.[21]

109. D. The blood flow within the terminal aorta in patients without peripheral arterial disease (PVD) is normally triphasic.[11]

110. A. The COS theda angle cursor should be placed parallel to the arterial wall or flow direction demonstrated in color to prevent the false impression of an increase in velocity.[5]

111. D. External landmarks cannot be found on every patient; therefore, an internal landmark such as a vascular common femoral artery bifurcation is preferred.[21]

112. D. There is a problem with the PRF aliasing occurring. The two sums are added to equal the total peak velocity.[5]

113. C. Color flow is essential for diagnosis of deep venous thrombosis (DVT) and the residual lumen in deep veins.[21]

114. B. Wall thickening is evidence that thrombus has existed in the past. Such veins become smaller as residual thrombus adheres to the venous wall, creating the impression of wall thickening.[21]

115. C. Many vascular specialists do not realize that the superficial femoral vein is a deep vein and requires treatment with any thrombus.[21]

116. D[28]

117. C. The arm pressure is compared to the calf pressure after the patient claudicates.[22]

118. C

119. A. A higher diastolic velocity occurs because of nonresistance. The internal carotid artery does not branch until it enters the brain.[5]

120. B

121. C. The common carotid artery most often can be dampened by severe proximal or distal disease or occlusion distally in the ICA.

122. B[20] (Courtesy of Benita Barthel, R.T., R.D.M.S., Ochsner Medical Foundation, New Orleans, Louisiana.)

123. A. Hepatopetal is the normal direction for flow into the liver; hepatofugal is the reverse out of the liver toward the spleen.[20] (Courtesy of Benita Barthel, R.T., R.D.M.S., Ochsner Medical Foundation, New Orleans, Louisiana.)

124. B. Reversal can occur with Budd-Chiari syndrome, cirrhosis, and right ventricular failure. There is no flow with an occlusion.[20] (Courtesy of Benita Barthel, R.T., R.D.M.S., Ochsner Medical Foundation, New Orleans, Louisiana.)

125. A[20] (Courtesy of Benita Barthel, R.T., R.D.M.S., Ochsner Medical Foundation, New Orleans, Louisiana.)

126. C[20] (Courtesy of Benita Barthel, R.T., R.D.M.S., Ochsner Medical Foundation, New Orleans, Louisiana.)

127. C[23] (Courtesy of Jeanie Marchese, Ochsner Medical Foundation, New Orleans, Louisiana.)

128. B. Values of .5 to .7 are considered normal.[23] (Courtesy of Jeanie Marchese, Ochsner Medical Foundation, New Orleans, Louisiana.)

129. C. The segmental artery is the most sensitive site for testing for renal transplant rejection.[23] (Courtesy of Jeanie Marchese, Ochsner Medical Foundation, New Orleans, Louisiana.)

130. A[23] (Courtesy of Jeanie Marchese, Ochsner Medical Foundation, New Orleans, Louisiana.)

131. C. The renal vein is anastomosed end-to-side to the external iliac vein. The renal artery is usually revascularized by an end-to-end anastomosis with the hypogastric artery.[20, 21, 23] (Courtesy of Jeanie Marchese, Ochsner Medical Foundation, New Orleans, Louisiana.)

132. C. Occlusion of the internal carotid artery is 90% accurate with color-flow Doppler technique. Transcranial Doppler and OPG are helpful in studying collateral circulation of the circle of Willis with internal carotid occlusion.[10, 23] (Courtesy of Dixie Alexander, Ochsner Medical Foundation, New Orleans, Louisiana.)

133. A[23] (Courtesy of Dixie Alexander, Ochsner Medical Foundation, New Orleans, Louisiana.)

134. D. Both the origin of the internal carotid artery and the carotid bifurcation are common plaque formation locations.[23] (Courtesy of Dixie Alexander, Ochsner Medical Foundation, New Orleans, Louisiana.)

135. C[23] (Courtesy of Dixie Alexander, Ochsner Medical Foundation, New Orleans, Louisiana.)

136. B. Tapping the area of the temporal artery with a finger may help to distinguish it from the carotid arteries. The temporal facial arteries dominate this region.[23] (Courtesy of Dixie Alexander, Ochsner Medical Foundation, New Orleans, Louisiana.)

137. A (Courtesy of Dixie Alexander, Ochsner Medical Foundation, New Orleans, Louisiana.)

138. B (Courtesy of Jeanie Marchese, Ochsner Medical Foundation, New Orleans, Louisiana.)

139. C (Courtesy of Jeanie Marchese, Ochsner Medical Foundation, New Orleans, Louisiana.)

140. A. High-resistance circulation is indicated in a typical Doppler waveform of the external carotid artery demonstrating a lower velocity in diastole. The facial and more superficial vessel branches create the resistance.[20, 23] (Courtesy of Jeanie Marchese, Ochsner Medical Foundation, New Orleans, Louisiana.)

REFERENCES

1. Bendick P, Glover J, Cornelius P. Noninvasive preoperative evaluation for placement of dialysis access shunts. J Vasc Technol 1992;16:172.

2. Bernstein EF. Noninvasive diagnostic techniques in vascular diseases. 3rd ed. St. Louis: CV Mosby, 1985.

3. Berry S, Sussman B. Determination of "good" saphenous veins for use in in-situ bypass grafts by real-time B-Mode imaging. J Vasc Technol 1988;12:184.

4. Carson PL, Adler DD, Fowlkes JB, et al. Continuous-wave Doppler and color-flow pulsed Doppler: relative sensitivity and breast tumor flow—a preliminary comparison. J Ultrasound Med 1992;11:S63.

5. Daigle R, Stavros T. Velocity criteria for differentiation of 60–78% carotid stenosis from 80% or greater stenosis. J Vasc Technol 1988;12:176.

6. Ellison J, Beach K, Cossman D, et al. Resting impedance measurements improves accuracy in plethysmography. J Vasc Technol 1987;11:227.

7. Fleischer AC, Rodgers WH, Kepple DM, et al. Color Doppler sonography of ovarian masses: a multiparameter analysis. J Ultrasound Med 1993;12:41.

8. Grant EG, White E. Duplex ultrasonography. New York: Springer-Verlag, 1987.

9. Hagen-Ansert SL. Textbook of diagnostic ultrasonography. 2nd ed. St. Louis: CV Mosby, 1983.

10. Kiell CS, Shepard A, McPharland M, et al. Efficacy of color-flow Doppler in the diagnosis of carotid artery occlusion. J Vasc Technol 1993;17:81.

11. Klemp K, Auer A, Blackburn M, et al. Detection of false aneurysm with color duplex scanning following percutaneous cardiac procedures. J Vasc Technol 1992;16:79.

12. Moulton-Levy D. Detection of renal artery stenosis by duplex and color-flow Doppler. J Diag Med Sonog 1990;1:1.

13. Neumeyer M, Gifford R, Thiele B, et al. Application of Duplex ultrasound color-flow imaging for the evaluation of renal allografts. J Vasc Technol 1991;15:156.

14. Nix L, Greenfield L. Duplex evaluation of inferior vena cava patency: a prospective study of patients with the Greenfield filter. J Vasc Technol 1987;11:167.

15. O'Leary DH, Polak JF. Interrograting the carotid with color-Doppler imaging. Diagnostic Imaging, November 1988;204.

16. Parker BD, Hallesey MJ, Rhall KS, Van Breda A. Noninvasive tests detect quantity and localize peripheral vascular disease. Diagnostic Imaging, October 1992;112.

17. Patin J, Singer J, Diserio F, et al. The identification of risk factors for deep vein thrombosis following major general surgery. The dyhydroergotamine/heparin multicenter trial experience. J Vasc Technol 1987;11:212.

18. Patterson R, Sullivan D. The effect of contralateral disease on carotid duplex accuracy. J Vasc Technol 1992;16:238.

19. Pellerito HS. Doppler scanning reveals physiology of transplants. Diagnostic Imaging, November 1992;132.

20. Rumack C, Wilson ST, Charboneau WJ. Diagnostic ultrasound. Vol 1. St. Louis: Mosby-Yearbook, 1991.

21. Rutherford R. Vascular surgery. 2nd ed. Philadelphia: WB Saunders, 1984.

22. Salles-Cunha S. Do claudicants have normal or decreased leg blood flow ratios at rest? J Vasc Technol 1992;16(5):241.

23. Sanders RC. Clinical sonography: a practical guide. 2nd ed. Boston: Little Brown, 1991.

24. Schroedter W. Delineation of lumenal contour in carotid arteries by color-flow Doppler. J Vasc Technol 1992;16(5):231.

25. Snell RS. Clinical anatomy for medical students. Boston: Little Brown, 1973.

26. Stephens T. Cardiac imaging correlates wall thickness with stroke. Diagnostic Imaging, March 1993;13.

27. Terry FM. Vascular scanning protocols. In: Tempkin BB, ed. Ultrasound scanning: principles and protocols. Philadelphia: WB Saunders, 1993.

28. Williams P, Warwick R, Dyson M, Bannister L. Gray's anatomy. 37th ed. New York: Churchill-Livingston, 1989.

29. Zweibel WJ. Introduction to vascular ultrasonography. 2nd ed. Philadelphia: WB Saunders, 1986.